"Ancestral diets and lifestyle practices have proven highly effective at curing migraines. Indeed, they are a general recipe for superb health and longevity. Josh Turknett has helped himself and many patients with these techniques, and now brings us the best available guide for overcoming migraines. If you have migraines, please read this book!"

—**Paul Jaminet, PhD**, author of *Perfect Health Diet* and editor of *Journal of Evolution and Health*

"I love, love, love this book. I personally suffer from an auto-immune disease, and this fun, easy read left me not only informed, but confident that I can live a longer life. As a chef, I found the diet and the recipes very achievable. Turknett really relates to everyday people in this truly informative and exceedingly helpful book. Life-changing."

—**Tracey Bloom**, chef, lifestyle consultant, Top Chef contestant, and co-owner of www.freecuisine.com

"Bold, eye opening, and compelling, *The Migraine Miracle* promises to forever alter the landscape of migraine treatment for the better. Essential reading for anyone who suffers from migraines, and essential reading for anyone who cares for migraine patients."

—**Timothy Lo, MD, MPH**, neurologist and pain management specialist

THE
MIGRAINE MIRACLE

A Sugar-Free, Gluten-Free,
Ancestral Diet *to*
Reduce Inflammation
and Relieve Your
Headaches *for* Good

JOSH TURKNETT, MD

New Harbinger Publications, Inc.

Publisher's Note

This publication is designed to provide accurate and authoritative information in regard to the subject matter covered. It is sold with the understanding that the publisher is not engaged in rendering psychological, financial, legal, or other professional services. If expert assistance or counseling is needed, the services of a competent professional should be sought.

Distributed in Canada by Raincoast Books

Copyright © 2013 by Josh Turknett
New Harbinger Publications, Inc.
5674 Shattuck Avenue
Oakland, CA 94609
www.newharbinger.com

Cover design by Amy Shoup
Acquired by Melissa Kirk
Edited by Marisa Solis

Library of Congress Cataloging-in-Publication Data on file

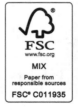
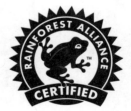

Printed in the United States of America

15   14   13

10   9   8   7   6   5   4   3   2   1   First printing

Contents

Introduction

I hate migraines.

No, really. I don't mean I hate *getting* migraines. It goes *way* deeper than that. I hate everything about them. I've spent most of my life hating them, in fact.

Growing up, I hated them because my mom had them. Hers were ferocious and frequent. And I couldn't understand it. One day she'd be fine. The next, she'd be fixing dinner or washing clothes, face pale and eyes squinting, trying her best to conceal from me and my brother the agony inside. She was never one to complain, never one to put her needs above those of our family. But I always knew, no matter how hard she tried to hide it. I could read her face as well as she could read mine. And I hated whatever could do this to her—these *migraines*, as she called them. I desperately wanted to help, but I knew deep down there was nothing I could do. She was the smartest person I knew, as knowledge-able about migraines as any doctor. If she couldn't tame this beast, then I certainly had no chance. Still, I would often dream of finding the answer, of one day making the discovery that could destroy it once and for all.

When I began getting migraines as a kid, I hated them with renewed vigor. I still vividly remember my first one—nobody forgets his or her first visit from the beast. I was eleven at the time, on an over-night trip with my school class. It was a trip I'd looked forward to all year long but barely had a chance to enjoy. Had I not seen my mom suffer with her migraines so many times I probably would've thought I was dying. I remember the bus ride home: the sound of the other kids having the kind of fun only kids on a bus can have, while I sat curled up in the fetal position in my seat, wishing they'd just be quiet, shielding my eyes from the skull-piercing rays of sun coming through the window. I got home, vomited until there was nothing left, and passed out in a heap of exhaustion. My life with the beast had begun. My mother's struggle was now mine, too.

Initially, my visits from the beast were few and far between. But as I got older, they came more often. By my thirties, I'd accepted migraines as an inevitable part of life. For as long as I lived, the beast would always be lurking nearby, ready to pounce after the slightest misstep. This was my fate, and I had accepted it.

Migraines still remain a family affair. As luck would have it, my wife also has them. Like my mom, she usually soldiers on in spite of them, sacrificing her own comfort for the sake of others. This means she knows what it's like to teach a room full of second graders with her head pounding, each tiny voice a cannonball crashing against her eardrum. She knows what it's like to twice spend the entire first trimester of pregnancy with migraines virtually every day, refusing to take so much as a single Tylenol. This kind of struggle takes its toll, though. It was hard enough for me to watch someone I loved go through it the first time around.

And when my daughter, at less than a year old, began having sudden episodes of intense vomiting, I wanted to believe it was just some odd stomach bug. But I knew better. I've known the beast long enough to recognize its many disguises. So it came as no surprise the first time she came up to me at age five with tears in her eyes and said, "Daddy, my head hurts." She was, of course, doomed by her DNA. Still, I didn't expect it to come so soon, though deep down I wasn't really surprised. I knew all too well that the beast shows no mercy.

So perhaps now you understand just what I mean when I say that I hate migraines. And perhaps it makes sense that I chose a career in neurology, the field of medicine that treats disorders of the brain, and thus bestowed myself with the task of treating migraine sufferers, or *migraineurs*. When I entered the field, there was a part of me that hoped it would provide me the opportunity to find the answer that could help my family, myself, and my patients cure their migraines and rid their lives of the beast. I learned everything I could about them from whatever and whomever—textbooks, journals, my teachers, and my patients. In spite of this, the ultimate cure remained elusive; but through these efforts I was at least satisfied in knowing I was providing my patients with every available tool for treating their migraines. It wasn't a perfect solution—in many cases far from it. But it was the best modern medicine had to offer, or so I thought. Ultimately I had come to the same conclusion my mother had years ago: the beast could not be killed; at best it could be *managed*.

But then it happened. In what seemed like the blink of an eye, everything changed. My migraine battle was over. And it happened by accident. Without intending to, I made the astonishing discovery that has completely transformed my life, that has completely transformed the lives of thousands of others, and that will completely transform yours. It is the discovery that will allow me to fulfill the promise I made to myself as a child so many years ago—my promise to kill the beast. At long last I've found its weakness, and the tool to exploit it. And I can't wait to share it with you.

CHAPTER 1

The Nature of
the Beast

Let's begin our discussion of migraines with a true account of one of my patients.

The Case of Margaret T.

Margaret T., an accountant in her late thirties, is usually fastidious about her appearance. Normally, she doesn't dare leave the house without makeup on, much less without taking a brush to her hair. But this isn't a normal morning. After having debated doing so multiple times during the past month, she finally drives herself to the local hospital, only to spend five agonizing hours under the harsh fluorescent lights of the emergency department's waiting room in order to earn less than five minutes with a doctor. To make matters worse, she leaves in basically the same shape she had come. Before she departs, a nurse hands her discharge paperwork with instructions to follow up the next day with a neurologist. This is the paper she hands to me when I walk into my exam room the following morning.

"Looks like you've been having headaches," I say.

"Yes, and they're awful," she replies.

"Can you tell me about them?"

"I get this pain, sometimes a dull ache in my forehead. But then it turns into this pounding pain in my left temple and around my eye."

"How long have you had them?"

"They started about a month ago."

"Have you ever had headaches like this before?"

"Well, yeah, I've had headaches before. I get sinus headaches sometimes. And sometimes I might get one from stress. But those are nothing like this."

"What do you mean by that?"

"Well, I've never had headaches this bad before, or this often. Usually I get a headache and I can take an Advil or some Tylenol and it'll go away after a while. But nothing seems to touch these."

"Nothing at all?"

"Excedrin helps a little bit, but I have to take it all the time."

"How often are you taking it?"

"Every four hours."

"You mean every four hours for the past month?"

"Yeah, pretty much."

"Yikes! Do you have any other symptoms with these headaches? Are you particularly sensitive to bright lights or sounds?"

"Oh yeah, I have to lie down in a dark room. And I can't stand for anyone to talk to me. I've also gotten really sick to my stomach a couple of times and thrown up."

Margaret hands me a copy of the brain MRI taken in the ER, clearly bracing herself for terrible news.

The above scenario is one that plays out in my office almost daily, and the conversation almost always travels along a similar path. Even for those who are well accustomed to migraines, visits from the beast can be frightening. For those who've never been visited before, their initial encounters with it are thought to surely signal the beginning of the end. But fear and anxiety usually turn to relief and even jubilation when they hear that not only are they going to be okay, but that—with a little effort—this beast can be conquered and destroyed.

Defeating the beast requires that we first understand its true nature. And when it comes to the nature of a migraine, misconceptions abound, both among the lay public and in the health care community. In this chapter, I'll cover just what a migraine is and is not.

PAIN WITHOUT A PURPOSE?

It's almost impossible for anyone to understand what it's like to have a full-blown migraine without actually experiencing it for him- or herself. And when you do experience your first full-blown migraine, it's almost impossible to believe that something isn't terribly wrong inside your head. After all, pain is supposed to mean something, right? It's supposed to signal that something has gone wrong inside your body so that you can then do something to fix it. When you step on a nail and your foot hurts, it's your brain's way of saying, "Hey, buddy, get that sharp thing out of our foot before we get a raging infection or bleed to death!" So a blinding pain inside your head must mean the same thing. Surely something terrible has happened in there. A rapidly expanding brain tumor, perhaps? A voracious brain-eating tapeworm? A ruptured cerebral aneurysm...or three?

Well, not quite. While those things can—and do—cause bad headaches on rare occasions (okay, maybe not the tapeworm), usually the cause isn't quite so exotic. This leaves me as a doctor in the difficult position of having to reassure my patients that, in this particular case, horrific pain occurred for no good reason. In this case, the pain wasn't a sign of something terrible happening inside their heads. And when they glance at me suspiciously while silently wondering whether I received my medical degree by mail order, I completely understand.

Yet, that's what I tell them. A migraine is not the sign of a sick brain. It is simply a process, a sequence of stereotyped physiological events that unfolds inside of otherwise normal, healthy brains. It's a mechanism that may result in a wide variety of symptoms, the most memorable of which is usually fierce, violent pain. But it's a mechanism that can be triggered inside anyone's brain, an extremely odd but "normal" physiologic reaction that occurs in response to specific triggers. Just a masochistic little glitch inside our brains, I say.

It's a hard sell. Trust me, I know.

THE MASOCHISTIC LITTLE GLITCH

A migraine is most easily understood as a process in the brain, a cascade of events that, once triggered, may result in a huge variety of symptoms, including numbness, tingling, visual disturbances, nausea, vomiting, dizziness, fatigue, and headache—a rich cornucopia of pain and suffering. This idea of a process unfolding inside our body in response to a specific trigger is a concept with which we're very familiar, as this kind of thing occurs inside of us all the time.

Take the case of a fever, for example. When our body is invaded by a microorganism, it is first recognized by ever-vigilant white blood cells whose job it is to detect intruders inside the body. This initial moment of recognition triggers a complex chain of events, one of which is the release of substances that raise our body temperature.

Or consider the swallowing reflex. When a bolus of food hits the nerve endings that supply the back of our throat, it generates a nerve impulse. That impulse then travels to the base of the brain, where it activates a highly orchestrated sequence of muscle contractions that propels food into the esophagus.

Both of these are responses we'd all consider to be part of normal physiology. Likewise, when the threshold for triggering a migraine headache is reached and the migraine switch is flipped, a sequence of events is set in motion in the brain, the result of which can be a wide variety of symptoms, including, most notably, a throbbing headache.

And though every last detail of this process is not entirely known, we've come quite a way in recent years toward understanding how it all happens. It's a complicated sequence with great potential for variation—variation that has resulted in a good bit of confusion.

The Glitch, Part 1: The Prodrome

The migraine process may be set in motion anytime from four to forty-eight hours before the actual pain starts, beginning with what is known as the *prodrome*. Not everyone experiences prodromal symptoms, and even those who do may only recognize their prodromal symptoms in retrospect. The most common symptom of a migraine prodrome is fatigue. In some, the fatigue can be overwhelming, and many may experience an overwhelming urge to sleep. Other reported prodromal symptoms include alterations in mood (irritability, depression, euphoria), food cravings, dizziness, diarrhea, constipation, and increased or decreased urination.

The Glitch, Part 2: The Aura

For many, the pain of a migraine is also preceded by an *aura*, a sometimes frightening but always temporary neurological disturbance that warns of an impending migraine headache. Auras are a sign that the migraine sequence has begun, that the beast has been roused and is on its way.

Auras may take many forms. In fact, virtually every type of neurological disturbance imaginable has been reported as a migraine aura. Visual disturbances are most common, followed by disturbances in sensation (numbness or tingling in the arm or face, for example). But, among other things, temporary disruption in speech, weakness in a limb, double vision, vertigo, or even complete quadriplegia have all been known to occur. The hallmark, though, is that these deficits in neurological function are always temporary, usually resolving after a period of about twenty to forty-five minutes. The experience of an aura, particularly the first one ever, can be terrifying. Not surprisingly, many folks worry that they are having a stroke, and, in fact, are commonly misdiagnosed by doctors as having almost had one (i.e., a TIA, or mini-stroke).

Back in 1941, a clever psychophysiologist and migraineur, K. S. Lashley, made a pretty remarkable discovery, and he did it simply through thoughtful observation and analysis of his own migraine aura. Prior to his headaches, Lashley would see what is known as a *scintillating scotoma*—a gradually expanding blind spot surrounded by crescent-shaped scintillations of light. This is, perhaps, the most common of all migraine auras. This shimmering blind spot starts out small, gradually enlarging in a predictable manner until it often ends up occupying half the field of vision. Using his knowledge of how the visual system is organized in the brain in combination with the observations of his own aura, Lashley reasoned that whatever process was occurring in his visual cortex to produce this particular phenomenon was spreading through the brain at a rate of two to three millimeters per minute.

In 1944, a PhD student at Harvard by the name of Aristides Leão made his own intriguing observation that seemed closely connected to what Lashley had described. Leão was studying brain electrophysiology using rabbits as subjects. What he found was that if he stimulated a rabbit's brain in any manner of ways—electrically, mechanically, chemically—he could elicit an expanding wave of depressed brain activity that spread outwardly from the point of stimulation. He calculated the speed at which this wave spread, and guess what answer he came up with? Two to three millimeters per minute. The exact same rate that Lashley had calculated in relation to his own migraine aura. That surely seemed like more than a coincidence.

Leão's experiment has since been replicated multiple times in multiple species. It's a physiologic response that, for reasons that aren't entirely clear, appears to be widespread in the animal kingdom—though we seem to be the only species in which it can be elicited without someone poking around in our brains. In recent years, we've developed technology that allows us to see this wave of depressed brain activity in real time during the aura phase of a migraineur, again always spreading at about the same speed that both Lashley and Leão described.

We now know that this wave of spreading depression in the brain is what causes the symptoms of a migraine aura. Most often, it starts in the back part of the brain, where visual signals are processed. This is why the most common migraine auras are visual in nature—flickering blobs, colorful fireworks displays, distorted objects, and the like. However, if other parts of the brain are affected by this wave of spreading depression, then different neurologic symptoms will occur. If the wave begins in the part of the brain that receives sensory signals from the skin, for example, then the aura may be a feeling of tingling and numbness on one side of the body. If it begins in the area of the brain controlling movement, the aura will be experienced as weakness in the arm or leg, or possibly even as problems with speech. Since virtually any part of the brain's cerebral cortex can be affected by this wave, virtually any type of neurological symptom may occur during a migraine aura.

Not everyone experiences auras with their migraines. Some folks may have one with every migraine, some may experience them occasionally, and some may never have them at all. Interestingly, however, it has been shown that at least in some migraineurs this wave of depression occurs without resulting in the subjective experience of an aura. Based on this finding, it is thought that perhaps there is some critical level of depressed activity that must be reached before the aura symptoms will actually occur. Thus, it is not entirely clear if this wave of spreading depression is a necessary feature of all migraines, either with or without the actual experience of aura symptoms.

Now we know a little bit more about all those funny symptoms that can precede a migraine. Fortunately, they're a lot less scary than they may at first seem. But we still haven't talked about why migraines hurt so badly.

The Glitch, Part 3: The Pain

The brain itself has no nerve endings, so it can't feel pain. I know, during a migraine it *feels* like your brain is hurting. But that's just a convincing illusion. In that case, then, where does the pain come from?

As it turns out, the surface of the brain is covered by several layers of connective tissue known as the *meninges*, which *are* entirely capable of sensing pain. It was once thought that the pain of a migraine was caused by dilated blood vessels inside this tissue. This was based on the observation that, after the wave of spreading depression ends, there's a temporary surge in blood flow to the brain—a surge made possible by expansion of the brain's blood vessels. It stood to reason, then, that it was this expansion of the blood vessels that was the source of the pain. More recent observations, however, show that the vessel expansion has long resolved even while the pain persists, and as such isn't likely the primary source of migraine pain.

Today, the prevailing theory is that the brain itself, or more specifically, the *brain stem*, is the primary generator of migraine pain. The brain stem sits at the base of the brain, forming the juncture between the brain and spinal cord. Normally, the brain stem is the *receiver* of pain signals. Pain-sensing nerve endings inside the meninges transmit nerve impulses from the meningeal tissue to the brain stem, which then sends it along to other brain regions that ultimately register it as pain. This is how an infection in the meninges (i.e., meningitis) leads to a headache, for example. In a bizarre twist, during a migraine, the signal direction is reversed: the nerve impulse starts in the brain stem and travels out to the meninges. This reversal of the normal nerve impulse direction is technically referred to as *antidromic conduction* (meaning opposite of normal), and is thought to be a critical early step in the generation of migraine pain.

Once that nerve impulse reaches the meninges, several different chemicals are released from the tip of the nerve (substance P, neurokinin A, and calcitonin gene-related peptide, in case you're interested). Among other things, these chemicals cause dilation of the meningeal blood vessels, spillage of protein from the blood vessels into the meninges, and meningeal inflammation. This inflammation then activates the pain-sensing nerve terminals in the meninges that then transmit the pain signal back to the brain stem.

Did you get that? The brain stem actually initiates the very signal that it ultimately receives back and senses as pain! If this sounds like a vicious, masochistic cycle, that's because it is! And this cycle continues, usually escalating in intensity until it finally burns out or something comes along to break it, like medication or a good night's rest.

The Glitch, Part 4: The Hangover

Anyone who has ever had a migraine knows that things don't just suddenly revert back to normal once the pain is gone. The brain—and the body—needs a little time to recuperate from the vicious sequence of events it just experienced. This period of recovery is typically referred to as the *postdrome*. Like the prodrome, fatigue or generalized "weakness" is the most common symptom reported. Some may also complain of "brain fog," or a feeling that they're just not thinking clearly. In addition, many migraineurs experience exquisite sensitivity in their scalp after the headache has subsided—the bristles of a comb may feel like tiny little needles raking across their skin. All of these symptoms can last up to a full day after the pain has subsided.

BUT WHY?

What I've described thus far is, in a nutshell, the migraine process as we currently understand it. I started by saying that migraines are just a physiologic reaction to certain triggers, just like a fever or swallowing. But there's just one little problem with this analogy: unlike a migraine, a fever and swallowing both have a *purpose*. Fever is our body's way of trying to destroy invading microorganisms with heat. And swallowing, of course, delivers food to the gastrointestinal tract for digestion. But what about a migraine? Spreading neuronal depression, antidromic conduction, sterile inflammation...*why* does this complex, highly orchestrated process happen at all? The truth is that nobody knows for sure. I have my own suspicions, which we'll discuss in chapter 4. First, let's talk about how we even arrive at a diagnosis of migraine.

MAKING THE DIAGNOSIS

There's no blood test, X-ray, or MRI scan that can diagnose your headache as a migraine. Despite all of the advances we've made in modern medicine, a migraine is still diagnosed the old-fashioned way: with a good patient history. In other words, the diagnosis rests on how you describe your headaches to your doctor. Sometimes blood tests and brain scans are performed as part of the evaluation for headaches, but this is only to exclude other, more exotic causes of headaches. These tests themselves can't actually diagnose a migraine.

So just what headache characteristics are considered diagnostic of migraines? According to the strict guidelines set by the International Headache Society (Olesen and Lipton 1994), migraines can only be officially diagnosed if you've had at least five headaches that meet the following three criteria:

1. The headache must last a minimum of four hours.

2. The headache must have at least two of the following four characteristics:

    *   a unilateral location (i.e., on one side of the head)

    *   a pulsating quality

- moderate to severe intensity
- aggravated by physical activity

3. The headache must be accompanied by at least one of the two following symptoms:

   - nausea and/or vomiting
   - sensitivity to light (photophobia) or sound (phonophobia)

These features describe a migraine in its most classic, fully expressed form. The good thing about these criteria is that if your headaches meet all of them, then chances are extremely high that you're having migraines. With criteria this strict and specific, the prospect of diagnosing a headache as a migraine when it is really something else is very unlikely.

The problem with criteria so strict and specific, however, is that rigid adherence to them would also mean underdiagnosing migraines by a large margin. In fact, I'd argue that if only those fulfilling these criteria were diagnosed with migraine, we'd be diagnosing the majority of migraine sufferers with something else. And without a correct diagnosis, we can't hope to provide proper treatment.

THE BEAST IN SHEEP'S CLOTHING

The reason why strict diagnostic criteria miss so many cases of migraine is because migraines come in so many shapes and sizes. As we've discussed, the migraine process consists of a number of interconnected events. It's a complicated process with many moving parts and many paths that may be taken once triggered. Furthermore, small and subtle differences in how those events unfold can translate to major differences in how the migraine is experienced. As a result, the migraine experience can vary greatly from one person to the next, and even from one migraine to the next in the same person.

With just the aura phase alone, the range of experiences is seemingly endless. As previously discussed, virtually every type of neurological deficit imaginable may present as a migraine aura. Likewise, the pain of a migraine, and the symptoms that accompany it, may also vary considerably from one individual to the next. Most folks, when they hear the term "migraine," will automatically assume this to mean a severe, throbbing headache. However, the pain of a migraine headache may range from mild to severe. In one migraine, dizziness and sensitivity to light may be pronounced, while the pain may be relatively mild. In the next, the pain may be excruciating and any ancillary symptoms minimal. Only when the migraine process unfolds in its most classic manner does it result in the prototypical migraine as described by the official diagnostic criteria—blurred or distorted vision followed by a severe, throbbing, unilateral headache accompanied by nausea, vomiting, and exquisite sensitivity to light or sound.

If we fail to recognize migraine in disguise, then we not only lose an opportunity to effectively intervene, we also oftentimes end up down a blind path that leads to wasted time, money, and effort. An isolated aura of transient weakness or numbness without any subsequent headache may lead to tens of thousands of dollars wasted on diagnostic tests for stroke—and quite possibly to unnecessary medications and procedures. A migraine with dizziness and nausea as its primary symptoms may lead to a fruitless search for inner ear problems. A diffuse, daily, moderate-intensity headache typically leads to months or years of anxiety over the prospect of a slowly growing brain tumor.

Because of this, it is quite common for a patient who has come to my office after having had his or her first prototypical migraine to have a longstanding history of episodic nausea, dizziness, malaise, fatigue, numbness, and so on. Most of the time, these symptoms have been ignored or have been erroneously attributed to something else. There may even be a long history of headaches that have been inappropriately categorized.

"SINUS" AND "TENSION" HEADACHES: FACT OR FICTION?

If you pick up a medical textbook on headaches and search the table of contents for "sinus headache," make sure you're in a comfortable spot, because you might be there a while. While the term "sinus headache" is ubiquitous in our popular lexicon, the actual diagnosis does not exist. How could this be, you ask?

It is believed the term "sinus headache" was first coined by drug companies selling medications for—you guessed it—sinus ailments. To help sell their medicines, they also sold the public on the notion that headaches that were accompanied by sinus congestion were "sinus headaches," and as such could be remedied by taking "sinus" medication. While this marketing effort has succeeded in selling a whole lot of sinus medication over the years, it hasn't helped too many folks with their headaches. In fact, it has likely done more harm than good.

The truth is, if we take the headaches most folks refer to as "sinus" and delve a little deeper, we find that almost all of these—around 90 to 95 percent according to several studies (Tepper 2004; Schreiber et al. 2004)—are migraines. It isn't hard to see why migraines are so easily confused with sinus problems. First of all, migraine pain is often around the face, including the area just adjacent to the nose, which most people think of as their "sinuses." And if the pain of a migraine is in the "sinuses," it seems reasonable to pin the blame on sinus problems. Second, migraines may also cause sinus congestion, and fluid may even drain from the sinuses just as it does during an allergic reaction or an infection. Combine pain in the area of the sinuses with sinus congestion and it's easy to see why the term "sinus headache" has had such staying power.

It is true that problems in the sinuses can cause pain. In the case of an acute, full-blown sinus infection from a virus or bacteria, there may be a sensation of fullness in the face, sometimes even pain or tenderness in the area adjacent to the nose. Because this occurs from an infection, fevers, chills, malaise, and sinus drainage will also typically accompany these symptoms, and the sinus area will also usually be tender to the touch. In other words, the source of the problem and the diagnosis in this case of sinus pain is typically obvious.

Further confusing the issue is the fact that a sinus infection or sinus congestion caused by allergies can often *provoke* a migraine headache. Migraineurs commonly experience a flurry of migraines in the midst of a sinus infection or during allergy season.

But is "sinus headache" overdiagnosis really such a big deal? The worst thing that can happen is that someone takes an innocuous over-the-counter medication that they don't really need, right? Could that be so bad?

Maybe so. First off, once we believe a headache has something to do with our sinuses, we're usually looking to figure out the cause. In this case, we're barking up the wrong tree, with no hope of finding what we're looking for. But besides the wasted effort, by mislabeling a migraine as something else, we miss opportunities to identify—and treat—what's actually causing our headaches.

Even worse, though, is that sinus medications aren't really so innocuous, *especially* when taken in the midst of a migraine. Not only do they offer little hope of relief for the headache, but the medications themselves—decongestants, antihistamines, and other sinus remedies, often used in combination—are notorious for causing what are known as *rebound headaches*. In a cruel twist of cause and effect, rebound headaches occur when the medication used to treat a headache starts *causing* headaches after repeated use—a vicious cycle for which the only solution is to stop the very medication you think you need. As it turns out, this is an extraordinarily common problem, most often caused by over-the-counter medicines. It's a problem we'll talk about in depth in chapter 4.

Almost as common as the notion of the sinus headache is that of the "tension headache." Headaches that are mild to moderate in intensity and not accompanied by sinus congestion or pain in the sinus area are often given this label. The idea here, which perhaps makes some intuitive sense, is that chronic "tension" in the muscles of the neck and face (usually attributed to stress) culminates in headache.

But, just as with sinus headaches, there's no plausible biological explanation for how this leads to headache. Sure, sometimes muscle tension or strain could lead to muscle soreness and/or tenderness in the muscles of the head and neck. But most people don't refer to this type of muscle soreness and tension as a "headache." In most cases, what folks with tension headaches are describing is migraine, once again in disguise. The situation is quite similar to sinus headaches. Just as migraines may commonly cause congestion in the sinuses, migraines may also commonly cause soreness or tenderness in the muscles of the head and neck. Furthermore, stiffness and soreness in these muscle groups are two of many factors that may trigger a migraine. Ultimately, however, the source of the actual headache is the migraine sequence unfolding in the brain. And, once again, effective treatment first requires correctly identifying the source of the problem.

THE GENETICS OF MIGRAINE, OR WHO'S TO BLAME FOR THESE THINGS?!

"But nobody else in my family has them."

This is one of the most common responses I hear from patients after they've been diagnosed with migraine. And it's a natural one. Most of us tend to categorize illness and disease as "things you can catch" or "things you get from your parents." We know that our family history has little impact on whether we'll get a runny nose from a cold virus or emphysema from cigarettes, for example. On the other hand, when we hear of a close relative having a stroke or cancer, we worry about how that impacts our own risk. Most folks tend to view a migraine as one of those things you get from your parents. From this perspective, then, it's reasonable to think that if they don't run in your family, you're unlikely to ever get one.

The truth of the matter is that most illness results from a complex interaction between our genes and our environment. The genetic material we receive from our parents may influence how susceptible we are to a given illness, but our environment can also tip the scales either toward or away from any given illness or disease. And migraine is no exception.

So while our DNA does matter, it's only part of the overall equation. Having a first-degree relative with migraines does indeed increase your tendency toward having them. On the other hand, not having any first-degree relatives with migraines in no way means that you cannot get them. The potential for migraines exists in everyone. As we've discussed, it's a physiological reaction that can be switched on at any given moment, in anyone. Where one person differs genetically from another is simply in how easily that reaction is triggered. Having a strong family history of migraine just means that, all other factors being equal, it's easier for the migraine switch to be flipped inside your brain compared to someone without a family history of migraine.

It's also worth mentioning that not knowing of a family history of migraine isn't exactly the same as not having one, for several reasons. One is that the general public awareness about migraines has risen considerably in recent decades. Therefore, people are more likely to seek medical attention for headaches and receive an "official" migraine diagnosis than they were in the past. Also, because migraine is so commonly misdiagnosed, many migraineurs may go through their lives not realizing that's what they have. Your brother's "sinus headaches" may have nothing to do with the pollen count. Those TIAs or "ministrokes" your uncle has been having all of his life may well be misdiagnosed migraine auras.

Lastly, there is usually more to our family histories than we realize. Quite often, my patients don't learn of a history of a particular medical problem or illness in their family until they're stricken with it themselves. Migraine is no exception.

That said, there are rare forms of migraines that do have very strong inheritance patterns. The most well known of these is *familial hemiplegic migraine*, a rare migraine variant whereby people consistently experience paralysis on one side of their bodies during their migraine aura, usually followed by a headache. Unlike typical migraines, whereby a heightened genetic susceptibility is conferred by multiple genes, in this particular form, the cause is a specific mutation in a single gene. The offspring of someone with these types of migraines has a 50 percent chance of having them as well. But this type of inheritance pattern is the exception to the rule, and families are usually well aware that this problem exists.

A migraine is simply a process that can be activated inside the brain. And just like a fever or swallowing, it's a process that exists within all of us. The only difference between someone who has frequent migraines and someone who rarely, if ever, has them is in how easily the migraine switch can be flipped. A strong history of migraine in your family is just one of many factors that brings you closer to flipping it.

THE IMPACT OF MIGRAINE

By now, you may be getting the idea that migraines are a lot more common than you realized. And you're right. Most epidemiological studies have estimated that between 10 to 15 percent of the US population has migraines (Lipton et al. 2007), and that number has been steadily rising in the recent past. That translates to around thirty to forty million people in the United States alone who carry a migraine diagnosis. That, by itself, is a staggering number, accounting for billions of dollars in lost productivity and innumerable hours of misery and suffering. In reality, for the reasons discussed in this chapter, the actual number is likely much larger than that. Clearly we're long overdue for a breakthrough.

CHAPTER 2

Crossing the Dreaded Threshold

After getting a prescription for sumatriptan, Margaret T., the accountant from the previous chapter, misses her six-week follow-up visit. Now, two years after her initial visit, she shows up again at my office.

"Hello, Ms. T.! It's been a long time! How have you been?" I ask.

"Well, I was doing great for a while. I took the sumatriptan you prescribed a couple of times after I was here the first time, and it worked great. And then my migraines stopped for a while."

"And now they're back?"

"Yeah, to say the least. They've actually been back for a while now."

"How often are they coming on these days?"

"They vary. Some weeks I'll have three or four days with a migraine. Other times I may go a week or two without one."

"Have you been able to identify anything that triggers them?"

"Well, yes and no. For a while I thought coffee was a trigger, but lately it seems to be helping when I get one. I know MSG [monosodium glutamate] is supposed to be a big trigger, and I feel like in the past I've gotten migraines from it. But just the other day I was starving and ate a bag of barbecue potato chips, and I didn't get a headache. And I used to be able to sleep in on the weekends with no problem, but lately I've been getting headaches when I do that. Sometimes they're bad during my cycle, but there are times I go through a whole cycle without one. Most of the time, though, they don't seem to be triggered by anything, they just happen."

LIFE ON THE EDGE

As miserable and debilitating as migraines can be, perhaps the worst thing about them is their unpredictability. If only we could know ahead of time when they are going to strike and for how long—then at least we could plan our lives around them. Not knowing if you're going to be out of commission from one day to the next is often what exacts the greatest psychological toll, leaving most migraineurs in a continual state of anxiety about when the beast will arrive next.

That's not to say we don't try to figure them out. Almost everyone who gets migraines with any regularity will try desperately to determine why they're occurring, in hopes of achieving some measure of control over them. But this process can be terribly frustrating. You may spend hours diligently logging your migraines, trying to detect any link between certain foods or lifestyle factors. And just when you think that you've got it figured out, everything seems to suddenly change. One day it may seem that almonds are your nemesis, and the next you find yourself eating them with no problem. Or, even worse, your migraines start occurring seemingly out of the blue. And, if that's the case, then what's the point of even trying to figure them out, right?

So why is it so hard? After all, the link between foods, lifestyle factors, and migraines is well established. In that case, it should be a straightforward matter of keeping a diary, pinpointing the trigger for each migraine, and avoiding those things like the plague. Yet many migraineurs do exactly this and still continue to suffer. So, what gives?

EVERYTHING MATTERS

Much of the confusion about what triggers a migraine centers around the popular misconception that each migraine attack is caused by *one* thing, and that those things are individual—in other words, what causes *my* migraines may be very different from what causes *your* migraines, as this line of thinking goes. Because of this misleading notion, many migraineurs end up looking for that *one thing* that caused each and every headache. If they consumed some MSG-laden Chinese take-out or drank red wine with dinner, they'll chalk it up to that. But what of all the headaches that occurred for seemingly no good reason, with no clear cause? And what of those nights they consumed a few glasses of red wine and woke up feeling fine the next morning?

With rare exception, it never really is any one thing that causes a migraine. On the contrary, when the migraine threshold is crossed and the migraine mechanism switched on, it's the culmination of many factors that gets us there. At any given moment, your migraine risk level is determined by the net result of all the things that both bring you closer to and farther from your migraine threshold. Once your risk level reaches that threshold, the migraine switch is flipped and the mechanism unfolds. Our ultimate goal, then, is to never reach that threshold, so that we never have a migraine.

To help you visualize how this works, imagine that you're flying in a basket attached to multiple helium-filled balloons. If you add more balloons to your basket, you ascend to a higher altitude. If you add weight to your basket, on the other hand, you descend to a lower one (for the sake of this exercise, just imagine you have a supply of balloons and weights you can add as you fly). At any given moment, then, the height at which you're flying is determined by:

1. The number and size of the balloons pulling you up, and

2. The amount of weight pulling you down.

Now imagine that if you reach an altitude of two thousand feet— your threshold—your basket will explode into a ball of flames (figure 2a). You don't want to do that.

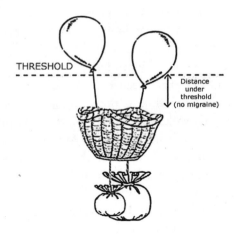

Figure 2a: Imagine that you are floating in this basket. The dotted line is your migraine threshold. At any given moment, the height at which you're flying is determined by the number and size of the balloons pulling you up and the number and size of the weights pulling you down. Cross the threshold and you rouse the beast.

Now let's see how this imaginary flying balloon relates to migraines. In this particular analogy, the height at which you're flying at any given moment represents your current migraine risk level. It is the net sum of all the factors that bring you closer to (the balloons) and farther from (the weights) the migraine threshold. Just as our flying balloon explodes when it crosses two thousand feet, so does your head when your migraine risk level crosses the threshold.

If our goal is to never allow our migraine risk level to cross the threshold, then it is critical that we understand the factors that raise and lower that level.

THE BALLOONS: BRINGING YOU CLOSER TO THE THRESHOLD

In this section, we'll cover all the factors that increase your chances of being stricken with a migraine. These are the balloons that pull up our imaginary basket. Any time you add a balloon, you raise your migraine risk level. Some items tend to raise your risk level more than others, and so I'll make note of the size of each balloon to reflect this. Small balloons raise your risk level a little bit, big balloons raise it a lot.

Fixed, Non-Modifiable Factors

Not everything that raises our migraine risk level is within our control. Some of these factors are genetic, embedded within our DNA and part of the hand we're dealt when we're born. Others are environmental factors that we can't do much about.

BIOLOGICAL

1. Strong Family History

As discussed in chapter 1, having a history of migraines in your family, particularly in a first-degree relative, increases your chances of having migraines. It's only one factor out of many, however, and many migraineurs don't know any family members who have them.

Balloon size: large

2. Hormones

This one applies primarily to women. The hormonal shifts that occur just prior to and during menstruation have long been linked to migraines. In fact, some women *only* have migraines around the time of menstruation, often referred to as *menstrual migraines*. Likewise, the hormonal shifts that occur during pregnancy can be a potent trigger, particularly in the earlier stages of pregnancy. In fact, I have treated many women who have experienced migraines only during pregnancy. On the upside, migraines usually improve considerably toward the latter half of pregnancy.

Many women also experience worsening of their migraines with birth control pills (as do postmenopausal women on hormone replacement therapy). Some women can minimize this effect by changing to a low-estrogen pill, while others must find alternate means of contraception (when possible).

Balloon size: large (women only)

3. Sinus Congestion

As discussed in the previous chapter, congestion in the sinuses (either from seasonal allergic rhinitis or a sinus infection) can also raise your migraine risk level, often leading to the frequently misdiagnosed "sinus headache."

Balloon size: medium

ENVIRONMENTAL

1. Strong Smells

Any particularly strong sensation can raise your migraine risk level, but smells are typically the worst. Strong smells from perfumes, scented lotions and creams, organic solvents, or other man-made chemicals tend to be the worst offenders.

Balloon size: medium to large

2. Sunlight

Bright sunlight, particularly if coming in from an oblique angle (i.e., from your side window in the car), is a very potent trigger for some. Tinting your car's side windows can be helpful if this is the case (though make sure you get a note from your doctor to give to police officers when you're pulled over).

Balloon size: small to large

3. Changes in Barometric Pressure

Many migraineurs complain of migraines whenever there's an approaching storm. The mechanism by which this leads to migraines is thought to involve the related drop in barometric pressure. Scientific studies on this issue have been somewhat inconclusive, but the preponderance of evidence suggests that it is a legitimate one.

Balloon size: small to large

Modifiable Factors

Unlike the fixed factors above, these are the balloons that you can (for the most part) control.

DIETARY

1. **Alcohol**

Alcohol is one of the most potent triggers of all. This depends to some extent on how much alcohol you consume, and the amount by which it raises the migraine risk level varies from one person to the next. Some migraineurs may get by with a drink or two and be okay. For others, it takes just a few sips to send them over the threshold. But almost anyone will get a migraine if he or she drinks enough ("hangover headaches" are migraines). Red wine has the reputation of being an especially strong trigger, but I think this is largely undeserved. It's the amount of alcohol consumed, regardless of the source, which seems to be the most important factor in raising the migraine risk level.

Balloon size: large

2. **Caffeine (Coffee, Tea, Sodas, etc.)**

This is a tricky one. Many people with migraines find out that caffeine can help abort a migraine attack after it has started. In fact, several migraine medications, including Excedrin "Migraine" (as well as regular Excedrin, which is the same exact medication), contain caffeine. So how could something that helps a migraine also cause them? Well, if I told you we really knew that answer, I'd be lying, though I have my suspicions (more on this in chapter 4). But the fact remains that caffeine can both help the pain of a migraine after it has begun *and* raise your risk level when you don't already have one. To complicate matters further, the time of day when the caffeine is consumed also makes a difference. Many migraineurs may be able to tolerate a cup of coffee or two in the morning with no problem, but not later in the day. The effect of caffeine, then, is situational, which is what makes it so perplexing. Last, just to make things more complicated, caffeine *withdrawal* (i.e., when you suddenly stop drinking caffeine-containing beverages regularly) will often trigger migraines.

Balloon size: medium

3. **Chocolate**

This one is a little bit tricky, too. While chocolate is almost always on the list of common migraine triggers, the case with chocolate is complicated by the fact that some migraineurs *crave* chocolate during a migraine, after it has already been triggered. And if you end up satisfying your craving before the pain begins, it may *seem* as if the chocolate caused the headache. That said, there is sufficient evidence that chocolate can raise risk level, at least in some individuals.

Balloon size: small to moderate

4. Monosodium Glutamate

MSG is a chemical used to add flavor to all sorts of foods. It's a common ingredient in Chinese food, often used to enhance savoriness. Many restaurants will now state if they're a "no MSG" establishment—if you don't see this information posted anywhere, then it's worth asking for a dish with no added MSG.

MSG is also a frequent additive in processed foods. If you're buying something that isn't in the produce or refrigerated section (i.e., it's food that comes in a box or bag and can live in your pantry without spoiling for months on end), read the list of ingredients on the label. And be on the lookout for some of the common MSG aliases on the ingredient list, including glutamic acid, glutamate, yeast extract, sodium or calcium caseinate, or any type of "flavoring" (e.g. "natural flavor," "chicken flavor," "beef flavor," etc.).

Balloon size: small to large

5. Processed and Preserved Meats

Basically, any type of meat product that you can buy at the store and eat without first cooking it yourself is a risk (salami, pepperoni, ham, jerky, bologna, hot dogs, etc.). It's thought that the nitrites used in the preservation process are the culprits, which you'll find on the list of ingredients (either as "nitrites" or "nitrates"). Meats and other foods that are smoked will also raise your risk level.

Balloon size: medium to large

6. Cheese

In general, aged cheeses are the primary offender here. As a general rule, if it's a hard cheese with strong flavor, chances are it will raise your risk score. Softer cheeses usually are not aged and so are less of a problem.

Balloon size: small to medium

7. Milk

Milk can be a mild to moderate trigger for some. Generally, the lower the fat content, the greater the potential for migraine. Lower-fat milk has a higher concentration of milk sugars, which are the likely trigger here.

Balloon size: small to medium

8. Citrus

Grapefruits, oranges, lemons, and other citrus fruits and juices can raise migraine risk. These seem to be most problematic when they're consumed alone on an empty stomach.

Balloon size: small

9. Bananas

Some people cite bananas as a potent trigger. In my experience, however, any sweet fruit consumed on an empty stomach can cause a headache. Bananas tend to get blamed most often because they are one of the sweetest fruits. Also, because they are fairly filling, easy on the stomach, and take no prep work, bananas are a fruit people commonly reach for to satisfy their hunger (which migraineurs should not do).

Balloon size: small to medium

10. Onions and Fermented Vegetables

Onions, particularly when consumed raw, can raise your risk level. Fermented vegetables like sauerkraut also act similarly. Pickled fruits and vegetables may also pose some risk, though likely to a lesser degree.

Balloon size: small

11. Nuts

Nuts of all kinds, such as almonds, walnuts, pistachios, Brazil nuts, and even peanuts are a trigger for some people.

Balloon size: small to medium

12. Fresh Yeast Bread

Freshly made yeast-risen breads are a problem for some. Examples include fresh sourdough, bagels, doughnuts, pizza crust, and soft pretzels.

Balloon size: small

13. Artificial Sweeteners

Aspartame (NutraSweet) and saccharin (Sweet'N Low), by and large the most commonly used artificial sweeteners in diet foods and beverages, are the most potent triggers in this category. The other alternatives—sorbitol, sucralose, mannitol, xylitol—appear to only modestly raise risk level.

Balloon size: medium to large (aspartame and saccharin); small (others)

LIFESTYLE

1. Stress

This is the granddaddy of them all, the trigger that gets blamed most often, in part because it's such an easy target. Stress is pretty much ubiquitous in modern life. Who among us makes it through a day without at least a little stress? So it's not surprising that stress is frequently blamed, even at times when it may not be deserved. That said, it is clear that stress (emotional or physical) significantly raises your migraine risk level. For some, emotional stress also manifests physically as tension in the neck and shoulders, which, as discussed in the previous chapter, can also trigger a migraine.

2. Hunger and/or Large Swings in Blood Sugar

Skipping or delaying meals is a commonly recognized trigger. Almost anyone prone to migraines has experienced headaches in this situation. More than likely it's the large drop in blood sugar, which produces the feeling of intense hunger, that actually raises the risk level. I have many patients who come in after the first prototypical migraine who report a long history of "hunger headaches," another instance of migraine in disguise.

Whatever you do, do not respond to a hunger headache by eating something sweet! And I don't just mean candy or desserts. A sweet piece of fruit (apple, banana, etc.) is just as bad and will cause your headache to escalate quickly! I must have made this mistake a hundred times myself, always thinking that I'd just waited too long to eat something before I realized that it was *what* I was eating to relieve my hunger that was the problem.

Balloon size: large

3. Sleep/Wake Cycle Disruption

This is another big one. Any disruption in your sleep/wake cycle can significantly increase your risk level. For most, this will be sleep deprivation, whether due to a night or two of insomnia, staying out too late on a Friday night, traveling overseas to a new time zone, or caring for a newborn baby. But it's not just too little sleep that's a problem; too much sleep can also ramp up your risk level. For some, the price of sleeping in on a Saturday morning isn't worth it.

Balloon size: moderate to large

4. Dehydration

Dehydration, or a deficiency in total body water, is another common culprit. This most often occurs after spending a long day outside in the summer, or after exercising for long periods in the heat. This is partly how alcohol, through its action as a diuretic (which causes water loss through the urine), causes migraines. If you're going to be outside in the heat for a while, make sure to drink plenty of fluids. Water is good, but replacing those lost minerals is also important, particularly if you're a "salty sweater" (you'll know if you are). You can drink a sports drink, but the sugar in these may pose a problem. A better option is to take an electrolyte tablet (available over the counter or online), or do what I do—take a pinch of kosher salt with your water.

Balloon size: medium

5. Heavy Exertion

Prolonged, intense exercise is a powerful trigger for some, while it may be insignificant for others. Typically, this is a problem for high-level athletes who are training very hard. Former NFL running back Terrell Davis famously had to sit out part of Super Bowl XXXII due to a migraine.

Balloon size: small to large

6. Sex

A small number of migraineurs reliably experience headaches during or immediately after sex. If this is true for you, then avoid it at all costs.

Kidding, kidding. If you do find yourself in this situation, try taking an aspirin (1,000 mg) or ibuprofen (400–800 mg) prior to intercourse.

Balloon size: small to large

7. Frequent Use of Migraine Medication

Somewhat paradoxically, each time you take a medication to abort a headache you also end up raising your risk level, such that your chances of triggering another migraine are higher after the medication wears off than they were before you took it (all other things being equal). We'll discuss this phenomenon a bit more later in this chapter.

Balloon size: large

8. Medications

Besides estrogen-containing hormone medication, other classes of prescription drugs will also raise migraine risk level. It may not always be feasible to stop or switch to another medication, but I always recommend discussing your options with your doctor if you're taking one of the following:

- Asthma inhalers/bronchodilaters (albuterol)

- Over-the-counter stimulants, which are just caffeine in pill form (NoDoz, Vivarin)

- Prescription stimulants (methylphenidate, dextroamphetamine)

- Nitrates/nitroglycerin for heart disease

- Erectile dysfunction medication (sildenafil, vardenafil, tadalafil)

- Acne medication (isotretinoin)

This list comprises the major classes of medication for which the link to migraine risk is well established. That said, it is certainly possible for other medications not listed here to raise migraine risk level. Any time there is a noticeable increase in migraine frequency after the start of a medication, it's always worth a trial of medication withdrawal (under your doctor's supervision) to determine if it is indeed the cause.

Balloon size: small to large

9. **Depression**

Clinical depression and pain don't mix well, as each reinforces the other at both a psychological and physiological level. Not surprising, a significant change in headache frequency is a common sign of depression, either from major depressive disorder or a reaction to a traumatic life event (death, divorce, etc.). And it is virtually impossible to bring migraines under control if this isn't being addressed as well.

Balloon size: large

Overwhelmed yet? Quite a list, isn't it? It's little wonder, then, that migraines are so common. I can't say I know anyone who has no stress, never stays up late, never sleeps in, never misses a meal, never drinks a caffeinated beverage or alcohol, or eats chocolate or citrus fruits...you get the idea.

But, as they say, knowledge is power. Thankfully, we're able to draw upon the accumulated experience of millions of migraine sufferers. And with so many potential triggers, it would be almost impossible to figure all this out on your own. If understanding what raises your risk level is one half of the battle in taking control of your migraines, knowing what lowers it is the other.

THE WEIGHTS: KEEPING YOU FARTHER AWAY FROM THE THRESHOLD

In this section, I'll cover the factors that reduce your chances of a migraine. These are the weights that lower our imaginary basket. Any time you add a weight, you lower your migraine risk. Like the balloons, some of these things are within our control and some are not.

Fixed, Non-Modifiable Factors

As is the case with the balloons, not everything that lowers our migraine risk is within our control.

BIOLOGICAL

1. Favorable Family History

Just as a strong history of migraine in the family can make you relatively migraine prone, little or no history of migraine may protect you. If you have no family history of migraine, then it'll take more balloons than it would for someone with a family history to raise your risk level up to threshold.

Weight size: large

Modifiable Factors

Fortunately for us, there are things we can do to add weight to our basket and lower our risk of a migraine.

LIFESTYLE

1. Regular Sleep Schedule

Migraines don't like consistency, especially when it comes to sleeping and eating. Though it may seem a little boring, your brain will thank you for sticking to a regular sleep schedule.

Weight size: medium to large

2. Regular Eating Schedule

See previous factor. In addition to keeping a regular schedule (i.e., consistent from one day to the next), you also want to make sure that your blood sugar level is staying relatively stable throughout the course of the day. One way to accomplish this is to avoid skipping or delaying meals. The most effective method for achieving this will be discussed in chapter 5.

Weight size: medium to large

3. **Stress Management**

It's rare that I have a patient tell me that he or she has never had a headache in his or her life. However, on the odd occasion when I do hear this, it is invariably spoken by someone who has no family history of headaches and is extremely laid-back—someone who never lets the inevitable ups and downs of daily life upset his or her calm disposition. As the wise Greek philosopher Epictetus once said, "It is not the facts and events that upset man, but the view he takes of them."

Finding ways to effectively deal with the stressors in your life is critical to keeping your migraines in check. For some people, like those who never get headaches, this comes naturally. For others, it takes a great deal of work. There are many great techniques for stress management—talk therapy, meditation, exercise, hobbies—enough to fill several books. Don't be afraid to ask for professional help if you find yourself unable to adequately control your stress, anxiety, and worry. It's a critical piece in taking control of your migraines.

Weight size: large

4. **Breastfeeding**

Most women with migraines will experience a significant reduction in headaches, or even a total respite from them, while nursing. Perhaps this is to make up for early pregnancy, when migraines are oftentimes at their worst!

Weight size: small to medium

DIETARY

1. **Supplements: Vitamin B2 (400 mg daily), Magnesium, Butterbur**

These are several "natural" remedies sold over the counter (easiest to find at health food stores or online). Just about everything under the sun has been extolled somewhere as a remedy for migraines, but these three supplements have the most quality evidence supporting them (Holland et al. 2012). While the effects aren't typically dramatic, the risks are minimal. These will be discussed further in the next section.

Weight size: small

2. Avoidance of Dietary Triggers

If we avoid the things that raise our migraine risk level, we will keep ourselves farther away from the dreaded threshold. There are different ways to go about finding your biggest dietary triggers. Of all the dietary triggers discussed, alcohol (not to excess) is the one that's a major factor for just about everyone. As for the others, you can determine their impact in one of two ways. The first is to maintain a food and migraine diary, which you can download from www.my migrainemiracle.com. Each time you experience a migraine, record it in your diary and then consult your food log to determine if you've recently eaten any of the trigger foods discussed earlier in the chapter. If you have an iPhone or iPad, you can also download the Trigger Tracker app that I created to help you efficiently and effectively track and identify your triggers.

The other method, which requires a bit more willpower, is to eliminate all of the potential dietary triggers we've discussed and reintroduce them back into your diet one at a time. The benefit of either approach is that identifying your food triggers will likely lead to a reduction in your headaches if you adjust accordingly. The drawback is that, since dietary factors aren't the only things that raise your risk level, you may at times mistakenly identify a food item as a major trigger when your migraine was instead caused by something else (poor night's sleep, the fumes of cleaning solution, etc.). Later I'll talk about the most powerful and life-changing dietary modification of all.

Weight size: small to large

PHARMACOLOGICAL

1. Prescription Migraine Preventive Medication

Though many drugs are prescribed "off label" for migraine prevention, there are four medications available by prescription that have been shown to have some ability to lower migraine frequency during clinical studies. I'll discuss these in more depth in the section "Ending a Migraine Attack—Migraine Abortive Treatments," later in this chapter.

Weight size: small to medium

Now that you have an understanding of all the various factors that both raise and lower your migraine risk, let's look at a couple of sample cases to see our imaginary flying basket in action.

The Case of Jane S.

Jane S. first began experiencing migraines roughly twenty years ago while in her early teens. She has been to countless doctors over the years for them and tried many different treatments. Both her sister and father have migraines, and she has come to the conclusion that migraines are her fate and there's little she can do about them. She has them often, taking prescription migraine medication on average three times a week. Jane considers herself a "worrier," often finding it hard to let go of things that bother her at work or at home. Consequently, many nights she doesn't sleep well.

One night in particular, she stayed up late working on a presentation for work, and then spent the remainder of her night worrying about how it might go the next day. Instead of the usual seven to eight hours of sleep she typically needs, Jane only spent three restless hours in bed. The next morning she woke with her stomach in knots. She tried to choke down a little breakfast but only managed a couple sips of orange juice. On her way to work, she noticed a small shimmering blind spot out of her right eye. By the time she arrived at work, her head was throbbing and she was sick to her stomach. Knowing she couldn't miss giving this presentation, she pulled herself together just long enough to make it through, though it didn't go as well as she'd hoped.

Let's first consider Jane's migraine risk level the day and night before her big presentation. Look at figure 2b to see how Jane's imaginary flying basket looks at that point in time.

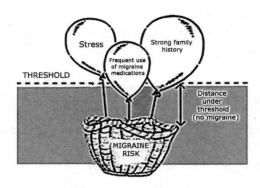

Figure 2b: On a typical day, Jane S. flies dangerously close to the threshold, thanks to stress, her frequent use of migraine medications, and her genetic makeup. In fact, Jane spends most days in the shaded gray area, always dangerously close to the onset of a migraine.

As you can see, because of her strong family history of migraines, her frequent use of migraine medication, and her near-constant state of stress and anxiety, she is never too far from her migraine threshold. In fact, as shown by the gray shaded area in the figure, she spends most of her life flying dangerously close to it.

Now let's examine how things look for Jane after her poor night's sleep and her glass of orange juice (figure 2c). Because she always lives so close to the threshold, these two factors easily propel Jane way beyond it and into full-blown migraine territory.

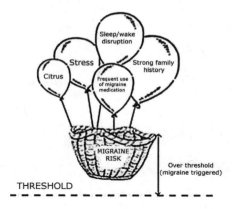

Figure 2c: All it takes is the addition of a glass of OJ and a poor night's sleep to take Jane S. over her threshold and into a migraine.

The Case of Joe C.

Joe C. is lucky. He's in his late thirties and has gone through his entire life never having a headache. He doesn't know of anyone else in his family who suffers from them either. Joe is a pretty laid-back guy. When things aren't going his way, he's able to let it just roll off his back. Nothing much worries him. Thanks to his favorable genetics and calm disposition, Joe spends most of his time (again represented by the shaded area in figure 2d) far, far away from the migraine threshold.

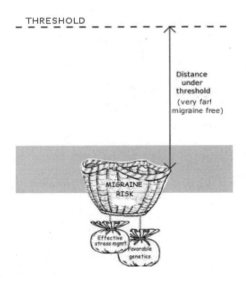

Figure 2d: On an average day, Joe C. is far from his migraine threshold, given his good genes and his even disposition.

But one week in particular proved a little different for Joe. That week, new neighbors moved into the apartment downstairs from him, and they're *loud*. The noise from their apartment (including the bass from their eighteen-inch subwoofer) usually crescendos around two o'clock in the morning. Since they moved in, Joe, who is normally a sound sleeper, has been sleeping about half as much as usual.

Worse yet, for the first time in years, Joe is finding work a bit stressful. His company downsized, and work that was once the responsibility of three people now falls on his shoulders. Furthermore, to counteract his sleep deprivation, he's been drinking about three times as much coffee as usual just to stay awake at work. Thankfully, Friday night arrives and Joe has the weekend off. Too tired to fix dinner or go out, he orders a pizza (sausage and pepperoni) and washes it down with a couple beers and a bag of nacho-flavored chips. The next morning he sleeps in. When he wakes up at 11 a.m. his head is pounding. It's unlike anything he's ever experienced. He takes two acetaminophen, then two more. Nothing. Head pounding, barely able to keep his eyes open, Joe hops in his car and heads to the hospital, convinced he's busted an aneurysm. Once at the hospital, he's sent straight for a CT scan of his brain. The scan comes back normal. The emergency room physician comes in the room and declares that Joe has just had his first migraine headache. Joe is skeptical. "But doc, I don't have migraines," he says, "and nobody in my family gets them either."

But Joe's doctor is right. Joe has just experienced his first migraine, a totally new (and frightening) experience. Take a look at figure 2e to understand how this came to pass.

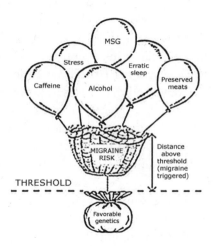

Figure 2e: After two weeks of poor sleep and stress, along with an uptick in caffeine, alcohol, MSG, and preserved meats, Joe C.'s balloons have carried him over his threshold, resulting in his first migraine.

For Joe, it required an almost perfect confluence of factors to bring his migraine risk level to the threshold. The point here, though, is that even in someone with no family or personal history of migraines, migraines can still strike at any time. However, because he spends most of his life far from his threshold, migraines never have been, nor will they likely ever be, a significant problem for Joe...provided he can do something about those downstairs neighbors!

THE ILLUSION OF A SINGLE TRIGGER

It should be clear from these examples that, although this remains a popular misconception, a migraine is never caused by any single trigger. Rather, it is the culmination of many different factors that together raise your migraine risk level above the threshold. It is easy to see, though, why the idea of a single trigger can be so convincing. To illustrate, let's take another look at Jane's case.

After finally recovering from her last migraine, Jane began to think back on it, trying to figure out just what caused it. She then remembered it began about 30 minutes after she drank that little bit of orange juice. She recalled a few other occasions when she had a migraine after some orange juice—and now she's confident she has found the answer.

The reality is that the orange juice probably had the least impact on her migraine risk level—it was just the final balloon that pulled her across the threshold. Convinced that this is it, however, Jane swears off orange juice, and in doing so neglects the impact of the stress, erratic sleep, and frequent use of migraine medication that will continue to maintain her risk level precariously close to the migraine threshold. Yet, were it not for these additional factors, that glass of orange juice wouldn't have mattered.

These cases should illustrate for you just how complex migraine behavior can be, and that figuring out the "cause" of any given migraine is anything but straightforward. Thanks to the single-trigger illusion, most migraineurs end up concluding that there are only two or three things that trigger at least *some* of their migraines, and these are what they end up trying to avoid. Furthermore, most migraineurs will have many migraines for which they are unable to isolate any trigger and end up reaching the conclusion that many of their migraines occur for no reason as all.

The truth is that all of the balloons and weights are relevant for everyone, and an awareness of how they affect your migraine risk level at any given moment is critical in gaining control over the beast. Avoiding every possible trigger isn't always feasible or practical, but knowing where you stand at any given time helps you make informed decisions. For example, if you've been particularly stressed out lately or slept poorly last night, then it's probably not the best time to have that glass of wine with dinner, since your risk level is already higher than average. On the other hand, if your menstrual cycle ended two weeks ago and you've been sleeping well, you may be far enough from your threshold that you can get away with that glass.

As a general rule, all migraineurs should aim to keep their migraine risk level as low as possible. We want lots of weight holding our imaginary basket down and very few balloons pulling it up. Later on, I'll discuss the most effective strategy for keeping your risk level far, far away from the threshold. First, let's talk about what you can do in those unfortunate occasions when you do cross it.

ENDING A MIGRAINE ATTACK: MIGRAINE ABORTIVE TREATMENTS

So, there you are, curled up in a ball in your bed, curtains drawn, head pounding, and you know you need to take something for your migraine. But what? The array of potential options, over the counter and prescription, is both a blessing and a curse. Make the wrong choice and you've just extended your headache by a few hours, if not a few days. And there are other factors to consider as well: cost, side effects, brand name, or generic. This is not the kind of multivariate analysis you're in any state to make in the midst of a full-on migraine. It can be an overwhelming proposition even when you're at your best. In this section, I'll review the available medications for migraine relief and simplify the decision-making process for you.

Over-the-Counter, "Nonspecific" Abortive Medications

Numerous over-the-counter medications are available for pain relief, some of which can serve as useful weapons in your migraine arsenal. All of the over-the-counter medications are considered "nonspecific" treatments, meaning that, unlike medications available by prescription, the mechanism by which they relieve pain isn't specific to migraine headaches.

ASPIRIN (BRANDS INCLUDE ECOTRIN, BAYER, AND BUFFERIN)

The original pain remedy, aspirin, classified as a nonsteroidal anti-inflammatory drug (NSAID), has been a go-to drug for pain relief for many years, and for good reason. It works, and it's cheap. Just don't go reaching for the baby stuff. Two extra-strength (500 mg each) aspirin offer the best chance of success, though they may be hard on those with sensitive stomachs. Frequent use may also result in a tendency toward bleeding and bruising.

OTHER NSAIDS (IBUPROFEN, NAPROXEN)

Inside the body, ibuprofen (brands include Advil, Motrin, and Nuprin) and naproxen (brands include Aleve and Naprosyn) relieve pain and inflammation in the same way as aspirin and as such are similar to aspirin in both their effectiveness in relieving a migraine attack and in their side-effect profiles. For migraine relief, the typical effective dose of ibuprofen is between 400 and 800 milligrams (two to four over-the-counter-strength pills), and between 220 to 440 milligrams for naproxen (one to two over-the-counter-strength pills).

ACETAMINOPHEN (BRAND NAME TYLENOL)

Though cheap and widely available, acetaminophen is not particularly effective against migraines. Those who do try it often end up taking more than the recommended dose in hopes of finding relief, which can put them at risk of liver injury.

COMBINATION THERAPY

As discussed earlier, the effects of caffeine on migraine are somewhat paradoxical. While in some instances it may raise migraine risk level and help provoke an attack, it is also well established as an effective remedy against migraine, particularly when combined with other pain relievers. It can be purchased over the counter, in combination with aspirin alone (brands include Anacin, BC Powder, Bayer Extra Strength Back and Body Pain, Bayer AM), or in combination with aspirin and acetaminophen (brands include Excedrin, Excedrin Migraine, Goody's, Pamprin Max, Anacin Advanced Headache). In my opinion, the acetaminophen is an unnecessary addition, again introducing the possibility of adverse effects while providing little to no additional benefit. As such, for those who respond well to combination therapy, I advise using preparations with just aspirin and caffeine.

It's also worth noting that you can create the aspirin and caffeine combination on your own. A great many migraineurs over the years have independently discovered that an "aspirin and a cola" or an "aspirin and a cup of coffee" is an effective migraine remedy. Should you attempt this approach, I'd recommend the coffee over the cola to avoid the blood sugar spike, as well as the other toxic effects of sugar we'll discuss in the next chapter.

SINUS MEDICATIONS

As discussed in the last chapter, some migraineurs experience pain in their sinus region (the area of the face adjacent to the nose) or sinus congestion during a migraine. Believing they're suffering from the fictitious "sinus headache," they reach for medication to alleviate sinus congestion.

These medications have no role in the treatment of migraine and, in fact, may aggravate the problem.

BRAND NAME OR GENERIC?

Standing there in the pain-relief aisle at the pharmacy can be overwhelming. Not only are there multiple brand names for each medication, most pharmacies have their own generic substitutions for each of these products. And they're oftentimes a whole lot cheaper! So what to do? Should you opt for the better bargain, or is this a case of "you get what you pay for?"

First off, there is no difference between the active ingredient in the generic or brand version. At the molecular level, aspirin is aspirin, regardless of whether it's labeled Ecotrin, Bufferin, or acetylsalicylic acid. There may be differences, however, in other aspects of the pills. Brand names are more likely to have an external coating of some sort, meaning they'll slide down the throat a little easier and can be gentler on the stomach. The rate of absorption between brand and generic formulations can also differ, which affects how rapidly the active ingredient enters the bloodstream. In some cases, this may spell the difference between success and failure. My recommendation, then, is to try a brand name first. If it works reliably for you, then try purchasing the pharmacy's generic substitute the next time. If generic works just as well, then you may end up saving a good bit of money in the long run. If it doesn't, you can just go back to the branded product and you'll only be out a few bucks.

Prescription Abortive Medications

For those for whom over-the-counter remedies are insufficient, a wide array of prescription migraine medications is available. Included within this group is the "triptan" family of medications, far and away the most successful class of migraine abortives ever developed.

MIGRAINE SPECIFIC: "TRIPTANS"

The year 1991 was a landmark for migraine sufferers. It was the year sumatriptan succinate (brand name Imitrex)—the first drug designed specifically to attack migraine physiology—was introduced into the marketplace. Sumatriptan binds to specific receptor subtypes for the chemical serotonin on the surface of blood vessels, constricting dilated blood vessels and reducing the inflammation around them. While ineffective for other types of pain, it is excellent at providing relief for migraines. In randomized clinical trials, 70 to 75 percent of those taking 100 milligrams of oral sumatriptan were headache free in two hours, compared with around 20 percent of those taking a placebo pill (Carpay et al. 2004; Sheftell et al. 2005).

For many migraineurs, my mother included, sumatriptan was the first medication that could ever abort a full-blown migraine. And it was a godsend. It was initially introduced as a self-administered injection, and not long afterward in pill form. Since that time, six other medications in the "triptan" family have been released. Like the original sumatriptan, they all work by binding specific serotonin receptors on cranial blood vessels. Their differences lie primarily in how quickly they're absorbed and how long they circulate in the blood.

Fast-Acting, Highly Effective Triptans (sumatriptan [100 mg], rizatriptan [10 mg], zolmitriptan [5 mg], eletriptan [40 mg], almotriptan [10 mg])

These five triptans, at the doses given, are the fastest-acting and most effective medications in the triptan family. They are also very similar in their potential adverse effects. Different insurance providers cover them differently, so choose the one that's the cheapest on your plan (i.e., the one with the lowest copayment). As of this writing, sumatriptan is the only triptan that has a generic formulation available, making it the most inexpensive option on many plans. In my experience, the generic (sumatriptan) is often just as effective as the brand name (Imitrex).

Slower-Acting, Longer-Lasting Triptans (frovatriptan [2.5 mg], naratriptan [2.5 mg])

These two triptans take longer to work and stay inside the bloodstream longer. Thanks to these properties, they are typically reserved for special circumstances. Since they're slower to reach peak blood levels, their adverse effects are typically less intense than their faster-acting cousins. As such, they can be a viable alternative for migraineurs who are particularly sensitive to triptan side effects.

Frovatriptan also has received special approval by the FDA for use as a preventative medication for menstrual migraines. When used for this indication, it is taken twice a day for five days, starting two days prior to the predicted onset of a woman's menstrual cycle. My patients have had considerable success using it in this manner, particularly those women who *only* experience migraines during menstruation.

Triptans Plus NSAIDs

For those who either don't respond consistently to a triptan alone or who only experience temporary relief, the combination of a triptan and a nonsteroidal antiinflammatory (aspirin, ibuprofen, naproxen) is a reasonable next step. These two medications have no significant drug-drug interactions and therefore can be safely taken together. The combination of sumatriptan and naproxen is available as a single pill under the brand name Treximet, which in clinical trials was shown to be more effective than sumatriptan alone. Insurance coverage for Treximet is variable, however, and you can replicate this combination on your own by using sumatriptan in combination with over-the-counter naproxen.

Triptans: Adverse Effects

For some folks (myself included), triptans may produce some mildly to moderately unpleasant sensations along with migraine relief. The actual feeling can be difficult to articulate, but is usually described as pressure or tension in the neck, shoulders, or jaw, or a feeling of "heaviness" in the body. These adverse effects are usually short-lived. They also are dose dependent, meaning they will be most pronounced when the drug is at peak levels in the bloodstream and will dissipate thereafter. Typically, these effects last for about 20 to 45 minutes. On the upside, the experience of these effects usually correlates with the onset of headache relief and thus some folks learn to welcome their arrival.

It's worth mentioning that these particular unpleasant triptan sensations are almost certainly a direct result of triptans' effects on the serotonin receptors on the surface of blood vessels. The same mechanism of action that produces migraine relief also produces the unpleasant sensations experienced by some. With this in mind, it should come as no surprise that, in general, the most effective triptans are also associated with a higher incidence of temporary unpleasant sensations. To remove these would require throwing the proverbial baby out with the bathwater.

Triptans and the Heart

As mentioned, triptans work in part by constricting blood vessels, leading some to worry that they may raise the risk of heart attack, stroke, or other "vascular events." At this time, this concern remains theoretical, as there is no evidence to date of any clear link between triptans and vascular events. Nonetheless, on account of these concerns, triptans are not typically recommended for those who have a history of heart disease, stroke, or uncontrolled high blood pressure.

Bypassing the Stomach

For some, nausea and vomiting is almost a universal feature of their migraines. When this is the case, orally ingested medications may not prove an ideal solution. For one, you run the risk of vomiting the pill right back out of the stomach—there's nothing more disheartening than watching an $80 pill float around in your toilet bowl. Furthermore, nausea is usually indicative of slowed transit in the stomach and gastro-intestinal tract, which may slow the absorption of the medicine into the bloodstream. So those who are in this predicament may require a route of delivery that bypasses the stomach. Fortunately, these alternatives exist. Sumatriptan, as mentioned, was originally introduced—and is still available—in an injectable form. The drug is injected subcutane-ously with a relatively easy to use "autoinjector," whereby it is then directly absorbed into the circulation. Both sumatriptan and zolmitrip-tan are also available as a nasal spray. Here, the drug is absorbed across the nasal mucosa and into the bloodstream, again removing the stomach from the absorption process.

MIGRAINE SPECIFIC: ERGOTS

The ergots ergotamine and dihydroergotamine are also considered migraine-specific medications, though unlike the triptans they weren't designed to be. Yet ergots are reasonably effective at relieving migraine pain, and, like the triptans, ineffective at relieving pain from other sources. Unfortunately, several factors limit their usefulness for most migraineurs. For one, *unlike* the triptans, they interact with multiple chemical receptors, creating the potential for a number of side effects, with intolerable nausea the most common. They are also not well absorbed orally, rendering the oral formulation a poor option. Nasal spray, suppository, and injectable formulations are available, though self-administration can be complicated. On the whole, then, it is the rare case for which ergots would be preferable to a triptan.

NONSPECIFIC: OPIOIDS

The oral opioids, which are all derivatives of the drug morphine, are nonspecific pain relievers. Due to their potential for habituation and abuse, they are also controlled substances. They are less effective than the migraine-specific agents at relieving migraine pain, and in many individuals may aggravate it. Beyond their potential for abuse, they also commonly cause sedation, nausea and vomiting, and constipation, and for most folks preclude work or social functioning for several hours. They also make driving unsafe. Since there are agents both over the counter and by prescription that are safer and more efficacious, they have very little usefulness in the treatment of migraine in all but the most extreme circumstances.

A Simplified Approach to Migraine Relief

This chart consolidates what we've discussed in this chapter into a simple and easy-to-follow process for choosing the most appropriate medication for ending a migraine.

Mild to moderate intensity, slowly evolving headache	>>	Nonspecific OTC medication (aspirin, ibuprofen, or naproxen), with or without caffeine (as a combination pill or with coffee)	>>	If not resolved in two hours or if symptoms progress rapidly, use fast-acting, highly effective oral triptan
Moderate to severe headache, or rapidly evolving symptoms	>>	Fast-acting, highly effective oral triptan		
Moderate to severe headache with nausea or vomiting	>>	Migraine-specific, non-oral formulation (injection or nasal spray)		

The Window of Opportunity

The difference between success and failure with any of the migraine abortive medications has much to do with timing. Generally, the longer a migraine lasts, the less responsive it is to abortive medication. As discussed in the previous chapter, a migraine is a chain of events that unfolds, in sequence, over time. The sooner you do something to disrupt that sequence, the better your chances of a favorable result. The longer you wait, the more likely that your window of opportunity will close. And, if you do find yourself (for whatever reason) having to wait a while to take something, it's best to go straight to a migraine-specific agent, ideally one of the fast-acting triptans.

Rebound Headaches

Earlier in this chapter, I mentioned that recent use of migraine medication can actually raise your migraine risk level, a phenomenon that seems paradoxical at first glance. On one hand, the medication may work to alleviate the headache you currently have, yet on the other it may make you more susceptible to another migraine in the near future—which brings us to the all-too-common problem of analgesic-overuse, or "rebound," headaches.

In the case of rebound headaches, persistent use of migraine abortive medication leads to a vicious cycle in which the drug both provides temporary headache relief *and* contributes to the recurrence of the headache once it wears off. It's a cycle that can continue indefinitely—I've known patients having daily headaches for *years* because of it. The only way to break the cycle is to stop taking the offending medication—a solution that may seem both counterintuitive and cruel. Though this varies somewhat from person to person, in general, taking an abortive medication more than twice a week greatly increases the risk of rebound headaches, yet another reason to find a way to stop migraines before they ever start.

MIGRAINE PREVENTATIVE MEDICATIONS

Speaking of stopping migraines before they ever start, what if you could take a medication every day that would prevent you from having a migraine, that could keep the migraine switch from ever being flipped on? For those with only the occasional migraine, it doesn't really make sense. But for those whose migraines occur weekly or more, it may seem like a dream come true. And in theory, such a dream is within the realm of possibility.

The reality, unfortunately, is not so simple.

As you might imagine, this is also an appealing idea to drug manufacturers. Not surprisingly, many drugs have been studied for their potential to prevent migraines. Of these, only four medications (topiramate, valproic acid, amitriptyline, and propranolol) have consistent, high-quality evidence demonstrating at least some ability to reduce migraine frequency. To do so, however, they must be taken daily. For most folks, committing to daily medication isn't something they take lightly. To justify such a decision, a migraine preventative must then fulfill two important criteria. It must

1. Work really, really well, and

2. Be virtually side-effect free.

So do our drugs meet these criteria?

The Case of Topiramate: Migraine Prophylactic du Jour

To see how the best available migraine preventatives fulfill the criteria we've given them, let's consider the case of topiramate (brand name Topamax), a drug viewed by many migraine experts as the best available migraine preventative available. Of the four most effective preventatives, it is also the one that was most recently introduced to the marketplace.

Topiramate is classified as an anticonvulsant, a medication to reduce seizure frequency in people with epilepsy. It works by suppressing the firing of brain cells, or their "excitability." It is thought that this is also how it suppresses migraine headaches. So how well does it work?

Several studies have been published on topiramate as a migraine preventative. Here we'll consider a typical one, published in 2009 in the journal *Headache* (Silberstein). In the study, 306 patients with chronic migraine headaches (more than fifteen headache days per month) were randomly assigned to receive either 100 milligrams of topiramate daily or a placebo pill. At the end of the study, those who had received topiramate on average had 5.8 fewer headache days per month than they were having prior to the study.

Sounds pretty good, right? At least until you consider that the patients who received an inert placebo drug on average had 4.7 fewer headaches per month.

In other words, taking topiramate every day only resulted in *one* fewer headache day per month than a side-effect–free sugar pill (and this in folks who were having *fifteen* or more headache days per month prior to the study). In the world of migraine prevention, however, where most drugs tested have no effect over placebo, this result, modest as it may appear, is considered an unequivocal success.

Yet, reducing headache frequency by just 19 percent compared to a placebo pill doesn't quite meet our criteria of working really, really well. Surely, then, topiramate, given its status as the migraine prophylactic du jour, must fulfill our second criteria of being virtually side-effect free. Right?

Unfortunately, side effects are quite common with topiramate. The most common is numbness and tingling in the arms and legs, a side effect experienced by roughly half of those who take it. Dizziness, sleepiness, nausea, loss of appetite, weight loss (not always unwelcome), problems with mood, and alterations in taste are also not uncommon. Perhaps most distressing, however, are the cognitive side effects that some experience: problems with memory, concentration, and word retrieval—effects that have led some to bestow it with the unofficial nickname "Dope-a-max" (a play on the brand name "Topamax"). Suppressing the excitability of brain cells has its price.

Are there any other prescription medications that fulfill our criteria any better? As mentioned, three medications besides topiramate—amitriptyline, valproic acid, and propranolol—are considered effective migraine preventatives. However, none have been shown superior to topiramate in reducing migraine frequency, and none are without their share of potential unpleasant side effects. Valproic acid, in particular, because of its potential for causing problems with fetal development, is not an option for women of reproductive age.

EXERCISE VS. TOPIRAMATE

In a 2011 study published in the journal *Cephalalgia* (Varkey et al.), researchers set out to determine how well a program of exercise fared against topiramate for migraine prevention. In the study, thirty-one migraineurs were randomly assigned to receive topiramate and thirty patients randomly assigned to exercise forty minutes per week (none of them were exercising regularly prior to the study). The exercise in this case involved a fifteen-minute warm-up, followed by twenty minutes on an exercise bike, followed by a five-minute cool-down.

During the three months of the study, those receiving topiramate experienced an average reduction in migraines of .97 days per month (i.e., slightly less than one day per month). Those who were on the exercise program experienced a reduction of .93 days per month. Exercise was just as effective as topiramate in preventing migraines—without the numbness, tingling, dizziness, taste disturbances, cognitive impairment, and so on.

THE CLINICAL TRIAL: REAL-WORLD DISCONNECT

As I'm sure you can gather based on this discussion, on the whole I'm not particularly fond of the migraine prophylactic medications, primarily because in my experience their marginal benefits are typically outweighed by their nontrivial risks. Yet they are promoted quite heavily by both the pharmaceutical companies and by professional organizations like the American Academy of Neurology, based almost entirely on their performance in double-blind, placebo-controlled clinical trials. For example, in a study based on survey data published in 2007 in the journal *Neurology* (Lipton et al.), it was estimated that 25 percent of all migraineurs should be offered daily prophylactic therapy, and the authors lamented the fact that only a relatively small portion were on these drugs. Indeed, upon initial inspection, the performance of migraine prophylactic medications in clinical studies can appear quite convincing. Yet, what practitioners like myself and patients have found, to their disappointment, is that the results realized in clinical trials never seem to accurately reflect what happens out in the real world of the neurology clinic. The improvements are often far more modest than what's reported in the study, and side effects are often much more of a problem than the paper would lead you to believe. Why might this be?

- **Artificial population:** Clinical trials are voluntary. Some folks will eagerly embrace the opportunity to be part of the testing of a new drug, while others find the idea of being a "guinea pig" objectionable. From the outset, then, the population in the clinical trial is not representative of the general population. Furthermore, once part of the clinical trial, participants generally want to see the study through to its conclusion. For multiple reasons, they want to be part of a trial that has a positive impact, and they want the drug to be a success. In migraine trials, these subtle biases, although well intentioned, may lead subjects to underreport side effects and exaggerate improvements. In the final trial analysis, all of these factors will tend to make the study drug appear both more effective and more benign than it actually is.

- **Placebo effect:** The placebo effect is very real and surprisingly powerful. Simply believing that a new treatment will help you can help turn that belief into a reality. This should not come as a great surprise, as it's entirely in line with our understanding of the relationship between the mind and body. Our thoughts, after all, are fundamentally rooted in biochemical changes in the brain. And given that the brain communicates with just about every part of our body, dramatic changes in our physiology can occur through thought alone—just ask the groom who faints in the middle of his wedding ceremony! Clinical trials do attempt to control for this effect, as typically half of all study subjects receive the active study drug and the other half receive an inactive placebo drug. Yet, the placebo effect itself is likely to be of greater significance for a patient in a clinical trial, as only those who believe it may be of benefit to them will volunteer for the study. Those who don't believe will never take part.

- **Augmented placebo effect:** Imagine you've had migraines for many years. You've tried several prescription migraine preventative medications and nothing has helped. Your headaches have gotten really bad lately, you're calling in sick to work more and more, and you worry whether things will ever get better (some of you may be able to relate to this quite easily!). Then you're in your doctor's office one day and she says that there's a brand-new drug being tested for migraine prevention. It's not yet available on the market, but you can enroll in a clinical trial and get it before anyone else. The only catch is that there's a 50 percent chance you'll get the actual drug and a 50 percent chance you'll get an inactive placebo pill, and you'll never be told which one you got. You decide to volunteer for the study and say a silent prayer asking to get the real drug. A few days after the study you start to realize that after every dose of the new medication your mouth gets a little dry and you feel a bit lightheaded—side effects! Hallelujah, you think, your prayers have been answered. You're taking the real stuff!

As mentioned, those who enter a study tend to be very hopeful about the prospects of the drug being tested—they *want* it to work. They are also usually thrilled to have the opportunity to be the first to have access to the latest thing that medical science has to offer. When those who are given the drug begin to experience side effects, they believe they've won the coin toss. The placebo effect is now kicked into high gear. Naturally, this will skew the efficacy data in favor of the drug. Yet this effect is in no way connected to its effect on migraine. Rather, it is an augmentation of the placebo effect and entirely an artifact of the clinical trial itself, not translatable to the real world of the medical clinic.

Unfortunately, migraine clinical trials are not designed to take the augmented placebo factor into account, nor are they required to. Research in the field of psychiatry, however, has shown the effect to be a powerful one. In several studies done decades ago on antidepressant drugs, researchers controlled for the augmented placebo effect by giving their subjects an active placebo, meaning it had discernible side effects. And the effect was quite impressive. On the whole, these trials showed that the benefits of the antidepressant medication being tested entirely disappeared when it was compared against an active placebo. Not surprisingly, the pharmaceutical companies are not too keen on testing for this effect when it comes to migraine preventive medications, and thus far the FDA has not required them to do so.

Botox

"You mean the stuff you use for wrinkles?"

This is the response I'm often greeted with after bringing up the option of Botox as a migraine treatment. To most folks these days, Botox is a cosmetic product. It's that stuff people inject into their faces to make them appear younger. Yet Botox wasn't originally developed in the name of youth and beauty. Rather, it was first developed as a therapy for neurological disorders that caused involuntary, and sometimes disabling, muscle spasms. Botox, a.k.a. botulinum toxin, is a muscle paralytic. When it circulates inside the body at doses that far exceed the amounts given for therapeutic purposes, it leads to the illness known as botulism. When injected into a particular muscle in very low amounts, it weakens it—a desirable effect if you have a muscle that is contracting too much. After Botox first hit the medical clinic, it didn't take long for folks to realize that it also helped reduce facial wrinkles if injected into the right spot.

Folks receiving Botox also started noticing that they were having fewer migraines. For many years, Botox neurologists used Botox as an "off label" treatment for patients with difficult-to-treat migraines. In 2010, after researchers confirmed its migraine benefits in placebo-controlled studies, Botox was approved by the FDA for use in patients with "chronic migraine," defined as having more than fourteen headache days per month.

Though I was initially quite skeptical, in my own experience using it in patients with chronic migraine, I have found it to be much more effective than the prescription migraine prophylactic medications. Furthermore, because Botox is injected directly into the muscles of the forehead, neck, and shoulders, it does not pose the same risk of systemic side effects as orally ingested medications do. Nor does it pose the same risk of drug-drug interactions for those taking multiple medications.

Botox's effects on the muscles last roughly twelve weeks, and as such most patients receive it on a twelve-week schedule. Although I always advocate dietary strategies as the primary means of eliminating migraines, I have found Botox to be a useful treatment for those unable to employ those strategies, or to help those with especially severe cases ease their transition to a dietary change.

Prescription Migraine Preventatives: The Final Analysis

To summarize, based on their lackluster effectiveness and potential for adverse effects, the prescription preventative migraine medications don't end up playing a worthwhile role in the treatment of most migraineurs, particularly when you consider that cheaper, safer, and equally effective means of migraine prevention exists.

Natural Remedies for Migraine Prevention

Though not as heavily studied as prescription medications, various medicinal herbs, vitamins, and minerals have been considered for their potential to prevent migraines, and a few have shown clear benefit in reducing migraine frequency.

Extracts of **butterbur**, a perennial shrub, have been used for various medicinal purposes for centuries. It has also recently gained popularity as a migraine prophylactic, and clinical trials have revealed that this is for good reason. In one randomized study (Lipton et al. 2004) butterbur (at 75 mg twice a day) reduced migraine frequency by 48 percent, compared with a 26 percent reduction for placebo.

Riboflavin, or vitamin B2, has shown similar effectiveness. In one study (Schoenen, Jacquy, and Lenaerts 1998), 59 percent of those taking 400 milligrams of riboflavin daily improved by at least 50 percent in headache days, compared to only 15 percent of those on placebo.

Multiple studies (Samaie et al. 2012; Gallai et al. 1992) have shown lower levels of the mineral **magnesium** in those with migraine headaches, naturally leading to speculation that magnesium supplementation could help with migraine prevention. And, while studies are limited, the existing data does support a probable effect of magnesium on reducing migraine frequency (Sándor and Afra 2005).

SO WHAT NEXT?

At this point, you now know virtually everything there is to know about the conventional approach to migraine management. If you're a migraine sufferer, this is valuable knowledge that you can use to reduce the number of migraines you get. It's knowledge that you can use to get rid of them more effectively when they come. It is the distillation of all the accumulated knowledge and experience I had acquired through my lifetime with migraines prior to 2010, both as a migraine sufferer and as a migraine specialist.

In the spring of 2010, though, everything changed. That was when I inadvertently discovered a way of reducing my migraine risk level more than I would've previously thought possible. It's an experience that has not only transformed the way I see migraine but that has transformed my entire life for the better. It can do the same for you.

CHAPTER 3

The "Miracle"

Prior to the spring of 2010, I thought I pretty much knew everything there was to know about migraines. After all, migraines had been a part of my life for as long as I could remember, my first exposure to them coming in my childhood as I watched my mother struggle mightily with them. And I also had my own personal experiences—and those of my patients—to draw from, not to mention the countless hours spent studying neurology textbooks and journals. Everything I'd learned from my life with migraines I applied toward my own care and to that of my patients.

With all of that accumulated knowledge and wisdom, I believed that I was doing the best job I could in managing my own migraines. I knew all the migraine triggers and had isolated the ones that were especially potent for me. Alcohol was a big one. Though I enjoyed doing so, I only rarely had a glass of wine or beer with dinner. And when I did, I'd chase it down with a few ibuprofens to mitigate the consequences, which still meant only reducing my odds of a full-on migraine the next morning by about half. I'd pretty much given up smoked or processed meats of any kind—sausage, pepperoni, or salami nearly guaranteed a throbbing head. Anything with MSG was also out of the question—probably a blessing in disguise since this meant almost complete avoidance of the snack-food aisle at the grocery store. I could eat nuts only in small quantities. A cup of coffee in the morning was generally fine, but definitely not after noon. Sleep deprivation virtually guaranteed a headache, yet that was hard to avoid when I was taking hospital call every fourth night. The one trigger that hounded me the most, though, was inconsistent mealtimes. As a physician, my schedule is usually dictated by how many patients show up for their appointments and whether I'm taking hospital call that day. Some days I would have enough time to grab a bite to eat for lunch, other days the mornings ran into afternoons with no break in between. Having a stash of protein bars helped, but on many occasions they just weren't enough. Driving home from work with a pounding head became a common occurrence.

I probably took medication for a headache roughly ten days a month, and maybe four of those days it was a triptan. Fortunately, my success rate with abortive medication was high, though it didn't come without a price. Taking a triptan generally guarantees a few hours' worth of overwhelming fatigue, often making the task of seeing patients or carrying out my responsibilities as a husband and father a bit of a challenge. But it was a price worth paying, as the relief from the migraine generally kept me functional—unlike the alternative. In my ten years since graduating from medical school, I'd only missed half a day of work due to a migraine. Knowing what I knew about migraines at the time, I thought that was pretty darn good.

So that's where I was. I'd accepted that my current migraine situation was about the best I could hope for.

Around the fall of 2009, while aimlessly cruising the Internet one evening, I happened upon a blog by a physician named Kurt Harris. It was a blog about nutrition that was written, oddly enough, by a neuroradiologist (a doctor who specializes in reading imaging studies of the brain). That, in and of itself, was a little intriguing. But it was the blog's main premise that really captured my attention. Dr. Harris argued that our current nutritional dogma—that a low-fat, low-cholesterol diet high in carbohydrates was best for optimal health—was dead wrong. Furthermore, our current dietary guidelines—the ones I'd been obediently parroting to my patients for the past decade—were resulting in a public health disaster, responsible in large part for the growing epidemic of diabetes, obesity, and quite possibly many of the other diseases we encounter most often as physicians. Harris advocated an entirely different approach to diet and nutrition, one that I ordinarily would have dismissed as patently absurd. But, try as I might to find reasons to reject it, I couldn't. In fact, it made perfect sense, despite the fact that it contradicted much of what I'd been taught in medical school. I realized that I owed it to my patients and to myself to dig a little deeper.

Let me first back up and say that, though this may come as a surprise to many folks, doctors-in-training receive very little formal teaching on the topics of diet and nutrition. In medical school, these are treated as an afterthought, as trivial and simplistic subjects that can be taught in the span of a lecture or two and that aren't particularly relevant to our jobs as physicians. Where I trained, we were basically told that there are two fundamental truths to remember.

One of these was that vascular disease, which is the proximate cause of heart attack and stroke, is best prevented by a diet that is low in fat and cholesterol.

The other was that obesity is caused by overeating and laziness. If you eat more calories than you burn, you get fat.

So we're told to tell our patients to eat low-fat foods and watch their calories. Done. Next subject. You'd think that something as important to human health as the stuff that nourishes our bodies day in and day out would receive a bit more attention. But, alas, most physicians view it as a diversion from more important things like ruptured spleens and exotic genetic mutations.

After reading Dr. Harris's blog, I came to the unsettling realization that I'd just blindly accepted that the dietary advice I was doling out to patients was built on a solid foundation. Like most doctors, I'd never actually done the necessary research to independently verify the information for myself. And I realized that was an unacceptable oversight, particularly for something so central to the health of my patients.

So then and there I decided, with my mind newly opened, to dive headlong into the field of nutrition. One of the first things I did was read Gary Taubes's *Good Calories, Bad Calories* (2007), a book that should be required reading for medical students and one I recommend to anyone interested in human health and nutrition. The book led me to revisit the finer points of biochemistry and endocrinology; to explore the epidemiological data on the link between fat, cholesterol, and heart disease; and to consider the subject from the fresh perspectives of human anthropology and evolutionary biology. Anything that could provide insight into what human beings should eat, I read. I was determined to unearth the truth in a field where it was often obscured by poorly conducted research studies with shoddily reasoned conclusions.

I'm not one to form opinions quickly, preferring to maintain an open mind and consider all points of view before forming my own. But when I emerged from this undertaking, I was disturbed. I was disturbed because what I'd been taught in school was so far from the truth. I was disturbed that my own personal vision of a healthy diet had been so misguided. I was disturbed that I had been unwittingly leading my patients astray for so long. I, along with the mainstream medical community, was giving patients dietary advice that was, without a doubt, worsening their health, unwittingly fueling the very diseases we are trying to fight.

Armed with this new information, I decided to make a change. And so, in the spring of 2010, with a renewed vision of proper nutrition, I overhauled my diet. I didn't do so to lose weight. I didn't do so to "feel better." I did it because my review of the research had led me inexorably to the conclusion that doing so would afford me the best chance of optimum health and well-being for the long term. Simply put, it would afford me the best chance to live a good life.

As it turned out, after making this change I did start to actually *feel* better. A lot better, in fact. The first thing I noticed was that I had more energy. The roller-coaster ups and downs in my energy levels I had assumed were an unavoidable fact of life were now completely gone. For as long as I can remember, I had always felt overwhelmingly sleepy after lunchtime and would struggle to make it through afternoons at work. Not anymore. I also noticed that my stomach no longer felt bad after eating. The indigestion I had considered a normal consequence of eating a big meal was gone. After a few weeks I also began noticing that the band of fat around my midsection, the "spare tire" that had been slowly building since high school, was starting to disappear. When the fat loss finally leveled off, my waist size ended up one size smaller than it was my senior year of high school.

As I said, I didn't necessarily expect any of this to happen, and I wasn't in this for weight loss, or to feel better. I was just eating the way I knew I should for optimal health. That said, these benefits were certainly a welcome surprise. But then, about a month or so into making this dietary change, I noticed something else…

I hadn't had a migraine. Not even a mild one. That was certainly noteworthy, but being the skeptic that I am, I still thought it was probably just a coincidence. Surely getting rid of migraines couldn't be this easy. I should know if it was, after all. I was an expert on the subject, for crying out loud!

Then two months went by. No migraine. Three months. Four. Five. Six...

Just like that, the beast was gone.

Not only did my migraines disappear, but many of the triggers that previously would've guaranteed a headache no longer triggered one. I started drinking a glass of wine with dinner. I could snack on nuts again. I could eat sausage or a plate of charcuterie. I could drink a cup of regular coffee in the morning—and in the afternoon. And those unavoidable lifestyle factors mentioned earlier no longer left me with a throbbing head. A sleepless night on call no longer meant needing an energy-sapping triptan to make it through the following workday. And, my erratic mealtimes—the trigger that used to plague me more than any other—were no longer an issue. I could go surprisingly long periods of time without feeling ravenously hungry, and, more importantly, without a trace of a headache.

Prior to the change in diet, I took prescription migraine medication on average between fifty to sixty times per year. In the year that followed, I took it once (when I "cheated" while dining out).

It's hard to convey how life-changing this experience has been. In fact, I wouldn't have believed it was even possible had I not lived through it. I had no expectation that any of this would happen with this change in my diet. But now that it has happened, there's no chance I'll go back to eating any other way.

And the best part? It can happen to you, too.

At this point, you may be wondering just what exactly led me to reframe my entire understanding of diet and nutrition. Why is it that I now believe that for the past half century or so we as a medical community have been doling out harmful dietary advice? To answer that question, let's start at the most natural place: the beginning.

REMEMBERING THE PAST

It's easy for us to forget just how long we human beings have been roaming planet Earth. Modern life is all we've ever known, and it's hard for most of us to imagine anything different. The truth, though, is that our current way of life, when viewed within the context of the history of our species, is really very new—a blink of the eye in the grand scheme of things. Based on archaeological records, our earliest human ancestors first appeared on this planet about two and a half million years ago. For most of that time, their lives were very different from the lives we lead today. And so were their diets. Our precivilized ancestors were hunters, eating the wild animals they killed and supplementing their diets when needed with the edible plants they foraged. Unlike our present-day societies, in which modern farming practices allow us to remain in one spot indefinitely, our prehistoric ancestors had to go where the food was. They hunted and they gathered.

During those two and a half million years, those who thrived on this hunter-gatherer diet passed their genes on to subsequent generations. Those who didn't perished, carrying their DNA with them. In this way, the human genome evolved over time, eventually becoming exquisitely well adapted to the diet of the hunter-gatherer. And while the environment most of us live in has changed dramatically since those days, the human genome has not. Our minds and bodies are still built for optimal function in a world we no longer inhabit.

It was about ten thousand years ago—a small blip in the huge swath of human history—that our way of life began to shift dramatically. This was the time when humans first began domesticating plants and animals, developing methods that allowed us to grow large amounts of food in one place so that we no longer had to roam the earth in search of our next meal. Humans could now stay in place for long periods of time. We were free to build civilizations, to develop technologies, and to write great poetry and music. Seen from this perspective, it's not hard to understand why this new way of life spread throughout the world. But as it did, our lives as hunter-gatherers faded away.

Though this transition was likely widely embraced as a sign of progress at the time, it did lead to some puzzling consequences. Body stature shrank considerably (Hermanussen 2003). Our brains got smaller. The average lifespan shortened. Skeletal remains reveal marked increases in the rates of tooth decay, iron-deficiency anemia, and other signs of widespread malnutrition (Angel 1984; Cohen and Armelagos 1984; Molleson 1994). In other words, after the advent of agriculture and continuing on until quite recently, we died earlier and were sicker while we were alive. You'd think that the stable food supply and lifestyle ushered in by the adoption of agriculture and pastoralism would've led to a healthier population. But these facts would indicate otherwise. How could this be?

An Unfamiliar Metabolic Milieu

Not only did the adoption of agriculture secure a more stable food supply, it also brought about a major shift in the types of foods humans consumed. The hunter-gatherer diet we'd been adapting to for more than two million years as a species, as well as the internal metabolic environment it created, had changed radically. It's certainly reasonable to think, then, that shifting to a diet we're not designed for could have an adverse impact on our health.

Then again, we're a resilient species. After all, we've been able to adapt to life in all four corners of the earth, so perhaps we could handle this dietary transition just fine. Is there any possible way to know what, if any, effect this change in the human diet has had on our health?

MODERN-DAY HUNTER-GATHERERS AND DISEASES OF CIVILIZATION

While most of the world transitioned from a nomadic hunter-gatherer lifestyle to one of farming and civilization, in some remote parts of the world there remained places where, even well into the nineteenth and twentieth centuries, the people did not. These remaining tribes of humans living, in many ways, like our Stone Age ancestors have afforded us a unique opportunity to observe what happens when humans transition from the diet of the hunter-gatherer to that of the modern human. The results aren't pretty.

Much of what we know regarding the health of these preagricultural populations comes from the records of colonial or missionary physicians, many of whom spent extended periods of time providing medical care for primitive societies on the African continent. In many cases, these doctors were able to witness not only the state of health of these groups as they lived a primitive hunter-gatherer lifestyle, but the ways in which the health of these populations changed as they *transitioned* to a modern, Western way of life—and a Western diet.

Time and again, the same story unfolded. In virtually every primitive society studied, from the indigenous peoples of West Africa to the Inuit in Canada and the Native Americans in the American Southwest, certain diseases were conspicuously absent. The disease whose absence received the most attention was cancer. In fact, its absence was so remarkable in the Alaskan Inuit, northern Athapaskans of Canada, and the native peoples of Labrador that it spawned a decades-long search among medical missionaries, anthropologists, and explorers to document just one case. They didn't succeed (Hutton 1925; Trowell and Burkitt 1981). Similarly, remarkably low rates of cancer—far lower than are seen now in the United States—were observed in Native American populations in both the Southwestern United States and northern Mexico (Hrdlicka 1908).

But it wasn't just cancer that was missing in these indigenous peoples. Several other diseases that most physicians today would consider "garden variety" were also glaringly absent, including diabetes, obesity, heart disease, stroke, asthma, stomach ulcers, appendicitis, arthritis, and gallstones (Trowell and Burkitt 1981). The ailments that now pay for a cardiologist's summer home on Cape Cod were nonexistent.

You might think, perhaps, that it was just because folks in these primitive societies, without access to modern medicines and sanitation, just didn't live long enough to acquire these particular diseases. But, on the contrary, the typical lifespan in these primitive societies was just as long as the nearby civilized populations where the ailments were commonplace (Hrdlicka 1908; Levin 1910).

Furthermore, an interesting thing kept happening as soon as members of these indigenous populations converted to a modern diet and way of life. Those diseases that were absent before the transition— diabetes, heart disease, cancer, stroke, obesity, autoimmune illness, dementia, gout, gallstones, and so forth—would invariably start to appear, usually during the span of a few decades. And they would consistently appear *together*, each time a population shifted from the diet of a hunter-gatherer to the diet of the modern postagricultural human (Trowell and Burkitt 1981), betraying their roots in a common cause.

Ultimately, these observations gave rise to the conception of a new category of illness—"diseases of civilization." These were diseases found in significant numbers *only* in civilized societies, begging the question of whether there was something about the life of a civilized human that was directly linked to their emergence. The one constant in all of these transitions was the change in diet. The agricultural revolution, the very thing that allowed humans to build civilizations in the first place, had also led to a major dietary transition—one that appeared to be making civilized humans sick in ways they never had been before.

Dr. Stanislas Tanchou, a French physician who systematically documented rates of cancer in death registries, was the first to present the idea that there were diseases unique to civilized life. He published his data in an 1843 paper in the journal *Lancet*, wherein his conclusion, later to be widely known as "Tanchou's doctrine," was that the incidence of cancer increased in direct proportion to the "civilization" of a nation and its people. Tanchou's findings were alarming—and a real cause for concern about the health consequences of our postagricultural diet. But the deteriorating health of hunter-gatherer societies after adopting a modern diet, and their relative freedom from disease prior to this change, serves as the most damaging indictment of our modern way of eating.

Much of this research on hunter-gatherer societies and the notion of diseases of civilization occurred toward the earlier part of the twentieth century. Sadly, much of it was neglected or ignored for a very long time. In fact, in my four years of medical school, I never once heard mention of it. I still find this hard to believe, especially given the implications of these observations for those of us entrusted with the public's health. Sadly, were it not for the medical community's ignorance of these findings, our current mainstream notion of a healthy diet wouldn't have ended up so embarrassingly wrong.

The Parable of the Wounded Animal

To frame this argument in slightly different terms, consider the following story. Imagine you're walking through the woods and you happen upon a honey badger with a wounded leg. It can't walk, and it's clear it won't survive long in the shape it's in. So, being the kind lover of nature that you are, you decide you'll take it home and nurse it back to health.

The problem is, when you get home you realize you have no idea what to feed it. At this point, you have two options:

Option 1: Scrounge up some items from your refrigerator and pantry, throw that into its cage, and hope for the best.

Option 2: Do a little research into the natural diet of the honey badger and feed it what it's meant to eat.

Which of these seems most reasonable to you?

The answer is obvious, isn't it? We all know that each and every species of animal has a natural diet—a particular set of foods it has adapted to and will function best on. If we feed an animal its natural diet, it should be healthy and thrive. If we feed it foods it hasn't adapted to eating, we know it will get sick. Most pet owners maintain strict control over the foods that their animals eat. I still remember the scolding I received as a kid when I offered some table scraps to my aunt's dog.

Yet, for some strange reason, we don't apply this same line of reasoning to our own diets. For the past ten thousand years, we've been eating foods that aren't part of the natural human diet, but most of us have never contemplated the possible health consequences. What comes naturally to us when caring for our pets we neglect when caring for ourselves.

Agriculture has allowed us to escape our ecological niche, removing us from the food environment our bodies adapted to and exposing us to one that's new and, in many ways, foreign. The diet we adapted to as a species isn't the diet we're eating, and it is making us sick. The overwhelming evidence on hunter-gatherer tribes and diseases of civilization clearly shows this to be true. It's remarkable, when viewed from this perspective, how we could have missed something so obvious for so long. Perhaps this oversight stems from our tendency to believe we humans hold some privileged place in the animal kingdom, that the rules that apply to "less evolved" species don't apply to us. Or perhaps it's simply because we've forgotten just how little time has passed in the course of human history since the end of the Stone Age. Whatever the reason, if we don't recognize and understand what has made us sick, we can't hope to get well again.

So what is it, then, about the civilized diet that causes disease? What is it in the foods we eat that leads to obesity, diabetes, cancer, heart disease, autoimmune illness, and so on? Well, if we know that something unique to our postagricultural diet is causing disease, then we should look at none other than the foods introduced by the agricultural revolution. So, without further ado, let's round up the suspects.

SUSPECT 1: CEREAL GRAINS

Any search for the disease-causing foods of our modern diet should logically begin with the cereal grains as the prime suspect, since without them the agricultural revolution would not have begun. Without cereal grains, and wheat in particular, there would be no pyramids in ancient Egypt. Without grains, Beethoven's Fifth Symphony would've never graced our ears. For better or worse, we owe civilization to grain.

Cereal grains are grasses of the monocot family that have been cultivated by humans so we can eat their fruit seeds. The most prevalent of these are wheat, rye, barley, rice, and corn, which together account for the bulk of calories that humans now consume. They're the main component of breads, pastas, cookies, cakes, pancakes, waffles, and breakfast cereals. All of these foods that most people eat every day were never eaten by our precivilized ancestors (Cordain et al. 2005). Without a doubt, this meteoric rise in grain consumption represents the most drastic shift in our food environment since the agricultural revolution.

Just why didn't our hunter-gatherer ancestors eat grains? Probably because they didn't want to die. In their raw form, grains are inedible, even toxic. In fact, most living things, including cereal grains, don't want to die—or be eaten. Just like you and me, all living things want to survive at least long enough to pass along their genes to future generations, and so throughout millions of years they have developed ways of discouraging other living things from eating them. Animals do this by running or flying away, hiding, biting, clawing, stinging, and so on. They can defend themselves from being eaten while they're *alive;* once dead, however, they are usually defenseless. Plants, on the other hand, can't run, fly, or bite, so they've had to devise other strategies to discourage other living things from eating them. The cereal grains' strategy is to make those who eat them sick.

Eventually, humans discovered that grains could be made edible by grinding them into a paste and heating them up. This was surely cause for great celebration, as a food source that had been unavailable for more than two million years could now be eaten. Furthermore, grains are packed with energy, can be grown in large quantities on relatively small plots of land, and can be stored for long periods of time without spoiling. In short, they are the perfect crop for sustaining civilization building, as they can support a large number of people in a relatively small area. Grain cultivation quickly spread around the world, ultimately becoming the cornerstone of the postagricultural human diet. No more hunting for our next meal.

But is rendering something edible the same as rendering it harmless, much less "healthy?"

Grain Problem No. 1: Nutrient Displacement

Compared to the nutrient content of most of the meats, vegetables, and fruits that composed the hunter-gatherer diet, grains are nutrient poor. They are an incomplete and inferior source of both micronutrients (essential vitamins and minerals we must obtain in our diets) and macronutrients (the carbohydrates, fats, and proteins that supply energy and support tissue structure).

MACRONUTRIENT CONTENT

All foods can be broken down into their relative amounts of the *macronutrients* carbohydrate, fat, and protein. Grains are mostly carbohydrate. If we consider one slice of whole-wheat bread, for example, we find it has 12 grams of carbohydrate, 4 grams of protein, and 1 gram of fat. In other words, 65 percent of the calories from a slice of whole-wheat bread comes from carbohydrate. It is a relatively poor source of protein, and a negligible source of fat. Since human beings can't survive without certain essential proteins and fats in our diets, we must get these from sources other than grains. As it turns out, of the three macronutrients, the only one we can live without eating *at all* is carbohydrate. You could live your entire life eating just protein and fat. Our bodies are completely capable of synthesizing carbohydrate, or, more specifically, glucose from other sources. This is not the case with fat and protein, as some amount of each is necessary for survival. So grains are an especially poor source of the proteins and fats we can't live without.

MICRONUTRIENT CONTENT

Besides protein, fat, and carbohydrate, foods also contain small quantities of various vitamins and minerals, also known as *micronutrients*. And when it comes to their micronutrient content, grains don't measure up here either. First of all, they don't contain vitamin A or C, both of which are critical to health and survival. They also lack vitamin B12 and contain negligible amounts of thiamine (vitamin B1), riboflavin (vitamin B6), and niacin. Devastating outbreaks of micronutrient-deficiency syndromes like pellagra and beriberi are not uncommon in developing countries where grains are consumed almost exclusively out of necessity.

Even in places where diets are more varied, the relative lack of nutrients in grains can create problems simply by *displacing* other nutrients. In other words, when we eat more of one thing, we tend to eat less of another. And so if we're eating a diet heavy in grains, as most folks do today, then it means we're eating less of the foods that are rich in the vitamins, minerals, proteins, and fats that our bodies need. Without grains, the multibillion dollar vitamin and supplement industry may never have had reason to exist.

Fortunately, many of us live in places where nutrient-rich foods are easy to come by. Most meats, vegetables, and fruits are superior to grains as nutrient sources. So what's lacking in grains can be found elsewhere. However, even when we do eat more nutrient-dense alternatives, the grains in our diet may prevent us from absorbing all that goodness.

Grain Problem No. 2: Antinutrients

As mentioned earlier, grains, like most other living things, don't want us to eat them and have devised several lines of defense to discourage us from doing so. Through modern methods of food processing we have weakened those defenses (or else we wouldn't be able to eat them at all). But, even with our best efforts, grains still put up a fight.

LECTINS AND LEAKY GUTS

Lectins, a family of proteins contained inside of most plants, are a primary plant defense strategy against predation. We still don't understand all the functions of plant lectins, but we do know part of their purpose is to discourage consumption by animals. And they do this by causing a host of unpleasant symptoms, or even death, in the animals who dare to eat them. Of all the foods composing the typical modern diet, grains and soy are among the highest in lectin content.

To understand what happens when we ingest lectin, let's consider the example of *wheat germ agglutinin (WGA)*, a lectin contained within wheat. Like other lectins, WGA is sticky, readily binding to other proteins it comes in contact with. After it enters our digestive tract, WGA sticks to the intestinal *villi* (fingerlike projections along the walls of the gut that are critical for the absorption of nutrients). The binding of WGA to the villi results in the damage and death of its cells. This destruction of the villi caused by lectins, including WGA, interferes with our ability to absorb nutrients from food. There is also evidence that lectins disrupt the gut's natural flora. These microorganisms in our gut not only play an important role in digestion, but their disruption can result in the growth and proliferation of unhealthy microorganisms, such as *E. coli*, which can overrun the normal gut microbial environment and make us ill.

In addition to interfering with the absorption of nutrients, the damage to the villi also disrupts another important function of our intestinal tract. Besides their role in nutrient absorption, the villi also provide a protective barrier between the inside of the digestive tract and our bodies. They control what comes into the body, and they also control what stays out. Lectin-induced damage compromises this essential role, creating what is referred to as a "leaky gut." Like a torn coffee filter, a leaky gut allows things into our circulation that aren't supposed to be there. Proteins that would normally be broken down into their composite amino acids before absorption end up entering the bloodstream whole. These proteins, recognized as foreigners by our immune system, ignite a chain of events that results in, among other things, the release of inflammatory substances inside the body as part of the body's efforts to destroy them. Furthermore, the presence of these foreign, undigested proteins also raises the risk of subsequent development of autoimmune illness (Cordain 1999)—one of the most well-documented diseases of civilization.

MINERAL-BINDING PHYTATES

Grains also contain significant amounts of *phytic acid*, or phytate, which is the form in which the mineral phosphorous is stored inside of plants. Humans lack the necessary enzyme to break down phytate, so it passes through our guts undigested. Furthermore, along its trip down our gastrointestinal tracts, it also binds to other essential minerals, including calcium, magnesium, iron, and zinc. Once bound, these minerals can't be absorbed into the body. Worse yet, the highest concentration of phytates are found in the whole grains we've been led to believe are so good for us.

Grain Problem No. 3: Foreign Proteins and Autoimmunity

Autoimmune illnesses, which include well-known ailments like lupus, rheumatoid arthritis, multiple sclerosis, Crohn's disease, hypothyroidism, and type 1 diabetes, occur when our immune system mistakenly mounts an attack against our own bodily tissues. In the case of rheumatoid arthritis, for example, the immune system attacks the joints, causing painful inflammation and deformity. In multiple sclerosis, the attack is waged on the nervous system, causing impairments in brain and spinal cord function.

Unfortunately, autoimmune illnesses are very common these days. You likely know someone with one or may even suffer from one yourself. And there is mounting evidence that many, if not all, of these are triggered by things we eat. To understand how this happens, let's first talk about the nature of autoimmune diseases.

In its mission to protect our bodies from invasion, our immune systems must determine what things inside the body need to be attacked and destroyed and what things need to be left alone. At the top of the list of things to leave alone is the body itself. It is critical that our immune system be able to distinguish friend from foe, and, for this reason, there's a complex system in place to accomplish this all-important task. Still, mistakes can happen. And those mistakes usually happen through the antibody-mediated immune response.

Whenever a foreign protein is encountered for the first time by certain white blood cells in our immune system, the system responds by producing an antibody to that protein. Once these antibodies are made, they can then bind to any of that particular foreign protein they encounter in the body, marking it for destruction and removal by other cells of the immune system. Viruses and bacteria have proteins on their surface, and antibodies that target these proteins are one of the primary means by which these unwanted organisms are eliminated from our body.

In some cases, however, a foreign protein may closely resemble one of the proteins in our bodily tissue. If a protein on a strep bacterium happens to closely resemble a protein in the heart tissue, for example, then the antibody made to combat that protein would result in an immune-system-mediated attack on the heart, which we know as rheumatic fever. In this manner, microorganisms may trigger an autoimmune illness long after the infection has resolved.

But it's not just the proteins in viruses and bacteria that can lead the body to attack itself. It is becoming increasingly clear that the proteins in our diet can also result in the same case of antibody-mediated mistaken identity and resultant autoimmune disease (Cordain 1999). And the dietary protein most likely to trigger this undesired response is *gluten*.

Gluten, a major component of wheat, barley, and rye, is a composite of two different proteins, *gliadin* and *glutelin*. Gluten is what gives bread its stretchiness and elasticity, qualities most folks enjoy. But gluten also makes some people seriously ill. It is estimated that about 1 percent of the population is gluten intolerant, though most are unaware of it. If gluten-intolerant individuals eat gluten grains, they develop what's known as *celiac disease*. Celiac disease is an autoimmune condition in which the gliadin protein in gluten grains generates an antibody-mediated immune-system attack against the intestines, leading to chronic diarrhea, fatigue, stunting of growth, vitamin and mineral deficiencies, anemia, nerve damage, and osteoporosis. Furthermore, those with celiac disease have higher rates of cancer, schizophrenia, and a whole host of autoimmune illnesses (Jackson et al. 2012; Rubio-Tapia and Murray 2010), suggesting that the body's response to gluten affects more than just the intestines. And, on the flip side, almost every chronic autoimmune disease we know of is associated with a significantly increased risk of celiac disease (Cosnes et al. 2008; Rousset 2004; Rodrigo et al. 2011; Song and Choi 2004).

But celiac disease is really just the tip of the iceberg. While 1 percent of the population is completely intolerant of gluten, it is estimated that a third of the population is at least gluten-*sensitive*, prone to manifesting a less severe form of celiac disease when exposed to gluten grains (Anderson 2012). And these gluten-sensitive individuals may suffer for years, if not their entire lives, with a host of unexplained symptoms, since few in the medical community are aware of how pervasive a problem this is. That fact alone should give anyone pause when considering eating gluten-containing foods. But, worse yet, the gliadin protein in gluten may well be the primary instigator of a number of other devastating autoimmune diseases. Not only does removing gluten from the diet cure celiac disease completely (Kneepkens and von Blomberg 2012), there is an ever-expanding number of anecdotal reports of folks who have reversed other autoimmune illnesses with a gluten-free diet.

Gluten was introduced into the human diet through the agricultural revolution, and it is becoming increasingly clear that most, if not all, of us were never meant to eat it.

Grain Problem No. 4: Carbohydrate Load and Fat Storage

As mentioned earlier, grains consist mostly of carbohydrate. This might not be a big issue if we only ate grains every now and again. But as the foundation of the modern diet, they make up the primary source of energy for most people. The typical American eats between 350 and 600 grams of carbohydrate a day, the majority of which is from grains.

It is our primary source of calories—in fact, the USDA food pyramid tells us this is the way it should be. However, it is estimated that our average preagricultural ancestors, thanks largely to the virtual absence of grains (and a few other modern sources of carbohydrate), consumed well under 100 grams of carbohydrate a day on average. That's a staggering increase.

Let's consider what happens to our metabolism when we eat carbohydrate, or, in particular, the carbohydrate in grains. Most of the carbohydrate contained in grains exists in the form of *starch*, which is just a large chain of glucose molecules. Starch is quickly broken down into its individual glucose units by enzymes in our saliva and those released by the pancreas. The glucose is then absorbed into the blood, causing a rise in "blood sugar."

The spike in blood sugar triggers the release of insulin from the pancreas, a hormone whose primary function is to remove glucose from the bloodstream by facilitating its transport into the bodily tissues. Once inside the tissues, the glucose can then be burned for energy. Once those tissues have their fill of glucose, however, any that's left over in the blood must still be eliminated. Glucose that stays around too long ends up sticking to bodily tissues and causing irreversible damage. So how does our body get rid of this excess glucose? It stores it…as fat. Yes, that's right. Any starch you consume that's in excess of what your body needs is, under the direction of insulin, converted to fat. And, in addition to driving the storage of glucose as fat, insulin also suppresses the release of fat from the adipose tissue.

So, in contrast to what you may have been led to believe, eating fat doesn't make you fat. Insulin is the primary hormone that drives the storage of fat in the fat tissues. And insulin is released not in response to dietary fat, but in response to dietary glucose. And the primary source of glucose in the modern diet is grain.

Now consider this: if 80 grams of carbohydrate were enough to support the energy demands of our hunter-gatherer ancestors—those same folks who roamed the earth on foot in a continual search for food—what do you think happens when a modern, sedentary human eats roughly five to seven times as much carbohydrate every day?

Hello, obesity epidemic. Nice to meet you.

Our meteoric rise in carbohydrate consumption has also triggered a meteoric rise in our insulin secretion. And, thanks to the metabolic effects of carbohydrate, we're not only storing more fat, but we have a harder time accessing that stored fat for energy (a topic we'll revisit more in the next chapter). So even though there's plenty of energy stored up in the fat tissues, in a high-carbohydrate diet it stays unavailable for use much of the time. In the naturally low-carbohydrate diets of our ancestors, energy needs were met largely by burning fat for fuel, which is why they were not obese. In the modern, grain-based, high-carbohydrate diet, our stored fat remains inaccessible most of the time. We must instead obtain our energy from the glucose in our next meal, and the cycle continues.

Grains: The Final Verdict

So the evidence is in, and the case against grains is substantial. Not only were they a negligible part of the human diet prior to the agricultural revolution, they have clear and plausible mechanisms by which they lead to the diseases of civilization. With other vastly superior sources of nutrition available and few redeeming qualities, grains (particularly those high in gluten and phytates) certainly are undeserving of their current status as an essential part of a "healthy diet."

SUSPECT 2: SUGAR

Sugar. Glorious sugar. Who doesn't love the stuff? It sweetens our sodas and makes doughnuts delicious. Few would argue that sugar is actually good for you, of course. It doesn't contain any vitamins or minerals, nor does it contain any protein or fat. It's just pure carbohydrate—a source of a little fuel for the body but otherwise nutrient free—just an "empty calorie," as they say. You certainly couldn't live on sugar alone, but otherwise it's pretty harmless. Right?

Prior to the agricultural revolution, humans didn't eat much sugar. Not that our ancestors didn't find it tasty, mind you, they just didn't have access to much of it. When they did eat it, it was in the form of fructose from the fruits they happened upon or, for those fortunate enough to live in the right spot, some wild honey. Estimates based on contemporary hunter-gatherer populations suggest that humans likely consumed around two to four pounds of sugar per year in our preagricultural days.

Now things couldn't be more different. Sugar is everywhere. The average American today consumes an almost unfathomable 150 pounds or more of sugar a year (USDA 2003). That's nearly a forty-fold increase over our hunter-gatherer ancestors. With an increase like that, we'd better be certain that sugar is nothing worse than a fattening "empty calorie."

Before we go further, let's briefly discuss what we mean when we talk of sugar. Table sugar, the white granulated stuff we buy in the large paper bags, consists of a molecule of *glucose* attached to a molecule of *fructose*. So it's half glucose, half fructose. High-fructose corn syrup (HFCS), which is also commonly added to foods for sweetness, is most typically around 55 percent fructose and 45 percent glucose. So for all intents and purposes, table sugar and HFCS are the same thing. Of that 150 pounds of sugar the average American eats, most of it is either in the form of table sugar or HFCS.

When we ingest either table sugar or HFCS, it is first broken down into glucose and fructose. From there, things proceed just as they did with the glucose from grains. Glucose in the blood triggers the release of insulin from the pancreas, and insulin drives the glucose into the tissues. What can't be taken up by the tissues is then stored in the adipose tissue as fat. Here again, it's not eating fat, but *sugar*, that is driving fat storage.

As for fructose, its metabolic effects are even more damaging. Unlike glucose, fructose can only be metabolized by certain cells in the body. In fact, the body treats fructose like a toxin, doing whatever it can to keep it out of the bloodstream. Like other toxins, the only place fructose can be metabolized is in the liver, where some of it can be burned for energy. What's left, however, is then packaged into triglycerides (fat) that are then released into the bloodstream. The more fructose we eat, the higher our blood triglyceride levels. Elevated levels of triglyceride in the bloodstream are a well-established marker of cardiovascular disease risk.

Another result of excess dietary fructose is that it causes fat deposits in the liver, just as it does in alcoholics. As such, it is referred to as "nonalcoholic fatty liver disease." And, like fatty liver from overconsumption of alcohol, fatty liver from overconsumption of fructose may eventually lead to the disruption of liver function and even liver failure (Tappy 2012; Abdelmalek et al. 2010; Lim et al. 2010). Fatty-liver disease appears to be a key component in the path to insulin resistance, the precursor state to full-blown diabetes (Smith and Adams 2011; Stanhope and Havel 2008). I don't think it's any coincidence that the epidemic of diabetes during the past few decades has occurred alongside the rise in sugar consumption during that same time frame.

Fructose and AGEs

Just what does happen if fructose gets into the bloodstream, if we ingest more fructose than our liver can protect us from? *Advanced glycation end products* (AGEs) happen. AGEs are formed when a sugar molecule in the bloodstream (like glucose or fructose) attaches to a protein on a cell in our bodily tissues (blood vessels, eyes, kidneys, brain, etc.). Once a sugar molecule sticks to a cell it disrupts its structure and function. *Permanently.* That cell will never be the same. In a diabetic, for whom the fundamental problem is an inability to clear glucose from the blood, these AGEs are formed throughout the body through the attachment of glucose to organ tissues. This is why the damage from diabetes is so widespread (heart, blood vessels, brain, nerves, eyes, kidneys). For those without problems clearing glucose from the blood, glucose-induced AGEs aren't as much of a concern.

Fructose, however, is *ten times* more likely than glucose to form an AGE when it comes in contact with protein. This means it would take a whole lot less fructose in the blood to cause AGE-mediated tissue damage and destruction. And the evidence continues to mount that AGEs are a path to disease in nondiabetics as well (Yaffe et al. 2011; Maillard-Lefebvre et al. 2009), again implicating fructose as the instigator of this damage. AGEs have been found in the pathological markers of a number of degenerative illnesses, including degenerative diseases of the brain like Alzheimer's and Parkinson's (Münch et al. 1998; Srikanth et al. 2011).

Fructose and Appetite

But, the bad news with fructose doesn't stop there. Fructose also plays an evil trick when it comes to appetite regulation. When sugar is consumed, the rise in blood glucose enhances the production of leptin, a hormone thought to suppress appetite in the brain. This is a natural and understandable feedback mechanism—your brain detects that you've just eaten some food, so you get the feeling that you're full. Fructose consumption, on the other hand, is associated with a *reduction* in leptin production. What this means is that, because of the effects of leptin in the brain, eating foods high in fructose may make you feel *hungrier*—in spite of the calories you've just eaten.

And, just when you think things couldn't get worse, there is also some alarming evidence linking fructose to cancer (Liu and Heaney 2011). We've already discussed the dramatic rise in cancer rates that invariably occurs after hunter-gatherers transition to a modern diet—one that includes a sharp rise in sugar consumption. However, even in postagricultural societies, marked rises in cancer rates have been repeatedly observed whenever *sugar* consumption increases.

The connection between cancer and sugar—and, more specifically, fructose—seems to stem from sugar's aforementioned capacity to cause insulin resistance. Once insulin resistance develops, the pancreas must release more and more insulin to clear glucose from the bloodstream. This is a good thing, on the one hand, in that it prevents blood glucose from reaching toxic levels (though ultimately leads to "pancreatic burnout" and the onset of diabetes). What's not such a good thing, though, is that cancer cells use insulin as fuel (Boyd 2003). The more insulin, the faster they grow. Obesity and diabetes are known to be associated with a major increase in cancer risk, and this may well be the reason.

So if insulin is cancer fuel, then we'd be wise to avoid the pathological elevations in insulin levels associated with insulin resistance. And how can we avoid insulin resistance? By avoiding sugar, the primary source of fructose in the modern diet. It is for this reason that, in a recent *New York Times Magazine* article by Gary Taubes (2011), two of the world's leading cancer experts confessed to being scared of sugar.

Sugar: The Final Verdict

Let's now consider the totality of the evidence on sugar. On the upside, sugar is very, very tasty. So tasty that we keep eating more and more of it, particularly if copious amounts of it are dissolved in brightly colored fizzy liquid.

On the downside, sugar is devoid of nutrients and is the quintessential empty calorie. It's also quite fattening, thanks to its knack for triggering the large spikes in insulin that direct it into the fat tissues for storage. Because of the unique way in which it is metabolized, it also causes fat buildup in the liver, leading to liver dysfunction and insulin resistance. As such, it may well be primarily to blame for the sharp rise in obesity and diabetes in recent decades, including the sad and unprecedented epidemic of obesity and diabetes in children we now find ourselves facing. Sugar consumption is also the primary dietary determinant of blood triglyceride levels, leading to the arterial plaques that result in heart attacks and stroke. And, last but not least, it may directly fuel the growth of many forms of cancer.

In a 2009 lecture entitled "Sugar: The Bitter Truth," Robert Lustig, University of California–San Franciso professor of pediatrics in the Division of Endocrinology and popularizer of the dangers of excess fructose, refers to sugar as a "poison." It's easy to understand why.

SUSPECT 3: OMEGA-6 FATTY ACIDS

If you've never heard of our third suspect, don't worry, you're not alone. But, rest assured, you've ingested plenty of it in your lifetime—certainly far more than our precivilized ancestors ever did. So what the heck is an *omega-6 fatty acid*?

To understand what omega-6 (also known as "n-6") fatty acids are, we must first understand fat. Fats, along with carbohydrates and proteins, are one of the three macronutrients. Though the misguided assault on fat that's occurred during the past few decades might lead you to believe otherwise, fats are actually critical to our health and survival. But not all fats are created equal, despite the fact that in popular conversation they're often talked about as if they are a solitary thing.

Fat exists in our foods in the form of *triglycerides*, a big molecule that consists of three fatty acids attached to a backbone of glycerol. Once inside our digestive tract, triglycerides are first broken apart by enzymes from the pancreas, which release the individual *fatty acids*. These fatty acids are then absorbed into the blood where they can be processed further. Our body first "sees" the fat from the food we eat as fatty acids. And it is the basic form and structure of these fatty acids that then determines their effects on the body.

All fatty acids can be categorized as either *saturated* or *unsaturated*. A fatty acid is "saturated" when all of its carbon atoms are attached to hydrogen atoms. It is fully "saturated" with hydrogen, in other words. Once a molecule is fully saturated, it is much less likely to react with things around it, because all of its attachment sites are full. This makes saturated fatty acids very stable, which is why they take a long time to degrade and have a long shelf life. An unsaturated fatty acid, on the other hand, has some carbon atoms that aren't attached to hydrogen, making them more likely to react with things they come in contact with. Within the class of unsaturated fats, we have both monounsaturated and polyunsaturated fatty acids. *Monounsaturated fats* have only one carbon atom that is not bound with hydrogen, hence the prefix "mono." As such, they are a bit less stable and more reactive than saturated fats. *Polyunsaturated fats*, also known as PUFAs, have two or more carbon atoms that aren't bound to hydrogen, rendering them the least stable and most reactive fatty acid species of all.

Omega-6 fatty acids, our third suspect, are a type of PUFA, and so are among the most reactive of the fatty acid species. Unlike our first two suspects, grains and sugar, we need some fat to survive. But, as with fructose, the problem here is in just how much of it we consume.

The biggest source of omega-6 fatty acids in our modern diet comes from vegetable and seed oils, which are a very recent addition to the human diet. You can't just squeeze some sunflower seeds or soybeans with your hands and get a jar full of oil. The oils must be chemically or mechanically extracted from plants or seeds—techniques that were only developed in the very recent past. Since our preagricultural ancestors did not possess the technology to extract these oils, the amount of omega-6 fatty acid they ingested was far lower than what the typical person eats today.

Linoleic Acid, Eicosanoids, and Inflammation

Besides being a fancy word good for impressing your friends, *eicosanoids* are also a large class of signaling molecules critical to our body's inflammatory response and immune function. They are made from the fatty acids in our cell membranes, and the particular fatty acid that is used determines the particular eicosanoid that is made. Eicosanoids that are made from an omega-6 fatty acid in the cell membrane end up eliciting a powerful inflammatory response, while those made from *omega-3 fatty acids* do not. As such, the ratio of omega-6 to omega-3 (also known as "n-3") in our cell membranes is a key factor in determining how many inflammatory molecules our bodies make. As a general rule, the greater the ratio of omega-6 to omega-3 fatty acids in our cell membranes, the greater the amount of inflammation in our bodily tissues.

So just what determines the omega-6 to omega-3 ratio in our cell membranes? Our diet. It is estimated that the diet of our preagricultural ancestors had a ratio of omega-6 to omega-3 fatty acids of around 1:1 or 2:1. Nowadays, thanks to the ubiquitous use of industrial-made vegetable and seed oils, that ratio is estimated at anywhere between 10:1 and 25:1. This distorted ratio then leads to the production of lots of inflammatory eicosanoids, and lots of inflammation.

This heightened state of inflammation is a big problem, as inflammation is a major component in a number of diseases including most, if not all, diseases of civilization. There is considerable evidence from epidemiological and animal studies that this distorted ratio, and the resultant heightened inflammatory state, plays a direct role in the development of cardiovascular disease, autoimmune illness, many forms of cancer, and mental illness (Simopoulos 2002).

So how can we save our bodies from this hyperinflamed state of existence? Simple: restore our omega-6 to omega-3 ratio back to what our bodies expect, which is estimated to be around 2:1. There are two ways we can go about doing this:

Option 1: Increase the amount of n-3 fatty acids in our diets. In other words, we can compensate for eating too much n-6 by eating more n-3, thereby restoring the ratio back to normal. You may have heard health authorities extoll the virtues of fish oil as a way of reducing your risk of heart disease, and this is why, as fish oil is rich in omega-3 fatty acids. The problem with this approach, however, is that omega-3 fatty acids are still polyunsaturated. If you recall our discussion on fatty acids, polyunsaturated fatty acids are the most highly reactive of all the fatty acid subtypes. This means that once inside the body they are very prone to oxidation (essentially a reaction with oxygen, similar to the reaction that causes an apple to brown when exposed to air), a process that leads to the generation of tissue-damaging free radicals. With this approach, though it's better than doing nothing, we're simply picking the lesser of two evils.

Option 2: The other, more sensible solution for restoring the omega-6 to omega-3 ratio is to simply reduce our consumption of omega-6 fatty acids. Not only does this return the ratio back to normal, it also keeps the overall level of reactive, oxidizing PUFAs in the body low.

A Brief Word on Trans Fat

In the mid-1980s, in one of the more devastating public health blunders of the past few decades, restaurants, especially those serving fast foods, were compelled to stop cooking with animal fats. This too was based on the unproven hypothesis that *saturated fat*—the primary fat in the lard used to cook French fries and other items—was a dietary evil to be avoided.

As a result, partially hydrogenated vegetable oils—things like Crisco and margarine—began replacing animal fat in restaurant cooking. A partially hydrogenated vegetable oil is one that has been chemically altered in a way that makes it behave more like animal fat. Through this treatment, oils that are typically liquid at room temperature are turned to solid, rendering them more stable and giving them some favorable cooking properties. The problem with partially hydrogenated oils, though, is that the chemical process also creates *trans fat*. Trans fat is a type of unsaturated fat that, as a result of the hydrogenation process, has a very unique three-dimensional structure. As it turns out, when these fats are incorporated into our cell membranes, this unique structure ends up wreaking all kinds of havoc—not at all surprising given that trans fats were not a part of the human diet prior to the past century. Trans fats have been linked to a number of diseases, including heart disease, obesity, diabetes, and cancer (Mozaffarian et al. 2006; Chajès et al. 2008; Stender and Dyerberg 2004). Fortunately, even the mainstream health community has recognized their dangers, and partially hydrogenated oils, once ironically enough considered the "healthy alternative" to animal fat, are now commonly viewed as a dietary villain. For once in the field of popular nutrition, common sense has prevailed.

If your food is coming from a chemistry lab, the safe bet is to leave it alone.

Getting Back on Track

The notion that animal fat clogs the arteries and that vegetable fats help to keep them clean has become almost as entrenched in our collective psyche as the idea that whole grains are part of a healthy, balanced diet. It's a message that has been propagated ad nauseam by the mainstream health authorities. For decades, the American Heart Association has told those with heart disease to substitute vegetable for animal fat whenever possible, a position initially adopted based on little more than a conjecture that animal fat was bad for the arteries. And it is a position that has endured for nearly half a century without any solid scientific support, and in the face of an increasing body of evidence that refutes it (Siri-Tariano et al. 2010). It is the foundation upon which virtually all of the mainstream nutritional recommendations have been built.

As it turns out, evidence continues to build that shows that the opposite is true. Not only does substituting vegetable for animal fat not protect against heart disease, it *worsens* it. This was laid out plainly in a study published in February 2013 in the *British Medical Journal* (Ramsden et al.). Sadly enough, the data actually came from a study that had been completed forty years prior. The paper itself was actually a reanalysis of recovered data from the Sydney Diet Heart Study that had been "missing" from the original report. The study originally took place between 1966 and 1973, involving 458 men between the ages of thirty and fifty-nine who had suffered a recent coronary event. In it, half of the men were told to substitute vegetable for saturated fat in their diets. In this case, they did so by using safflower oil, an especially rich source of omega-6 fatty acid. The other half, the control group, was not told to make any specific dietary changes. The results were a major blow to anyone still clinging to the notion that animal fat is bad for the arteries. In this study, those who substituted vegetable for animal fat were *35 percent more likely to die from a heart attack*, and 29 percent more likely to die from any cause. And this result was in spite of the fact that their total cholesterol levels were more than 20 points lower than those in the control group.

The *only* reason we've been told to eat less animal and more vegetable fat is because it's supposed to help us ward off the arterial hardening that leads to heart attacks and other problems. Not only is this an evolutionarily discordant piece of advice, this study reveals it to be entirely *backward*.

Though it should have been extinguished long ago, the belief that animal fat leads to heart disease is one that I am confident will ultimately die away. It is a notion that has arisen not from the rigorous application of the scientific method, but rather from a mix of hubris, bad science, and hasty public-policy making (Taubes 2008). Eventually, though, good science will prevail, and it will collapse under the weight of the scientific evidence against it. Once this happens, the landscape of mainstream nutrition will be changed forever for the better.

Omega-6 Fatty Acids: The Verdict

While small amounts of linoleic acids are necessary for survival, the current amounts eaten in the standard American diet create a heightened state of inflammation inside the body, contributing to the development of many, if not all, of the diseases of civilization. Contrary to popular belief, vegetable fat is not better for you than animal fat. And trans fats should remain in the chemistry laboratory, not in your pantry.

SUSPECT 4: DAIRY

Since the advent of agriculture and animal husbandry, humans have been raising animals not just for their meat, but also for their milk. For a complete source of nutrition, milk is hard to beat. Yet, for most of human existence on this planet, humans didn't drink the milk of other animals. For this reason, milk, or dairy in general, deserves consideration as another possible disease-causing agent in our modern diet.

Milk has a lot of things going for it. Unlike the cereal grains that have, through the evolutionary process of natural selection, developed specific strategies to discourage us from eating them, milk's sole purpose is to nourish an animal. It is designed to be the *only* source of energy and nutrition for a developing mammal. Not surprisingly, it contains all nine essential amino acids, is loaded with vitamins and minerals, and is a balanced source of carbohydrate, proteins, and fat. In many ways, milk is the perfect food. And humans have indeed been consuming a form of it—human milk—as long as we've been on this planet. In this sense, our genome has had a very long time to adapt to milk. It is only our consumption of nonhuman milk that is a relatively recent phenomenon. Thus far, there isn't any compelling link between nonhuman milk consumption and the diseases of civilization—likely because nonhuman milk is so similar to our own. However, while it doesn't appear to have anywhere near the disease-causing potential of the other suspects we've discussed, milk can create certain problems for some.

Milk and Lactose Intolerance

The naturally occurring sugar in milk is in the form of *lactose*, a molecule that's composed of one molecule of glucose and one molecule of galactose. In order for lactose to be absorbed, it must first be broken down by the enzyme lactase into these two components. If it isn't broken down, it instead passes into our gut intact, where it leads to bloating, gas, diarrhea, and other unpleasantness. All humans make plenty of lactase during infancy and early childhood, as our bodies expect to be running on the milk of our mothers. On the other hand, most of us produce less lactase as we get older, though how much less depends in large part on ethnic background. Those of African and Asian descent tend to produce the least, while those of Northern European ancestry may never reduce their lactase production at all. Lactose intolerance isn't typically subtle—those who have it are often quite uncomfortable after consuming dairy that's high in lactose. Fermented dairy products like yogurt and cheese have very low amounts of lactose and are usually tolerated just fine by those with lactose intolerance, however.

Milk Allergy

Casein is a class of proteins that are found in milk. The type of casein found varies by species, so the casein found in cows is different than that found in humans. For a small number of people, this difference in casein protein composition can result in an allergic reaction. The reaction can be extreme, with symptoms including wheezing, hives, and vomiting. It occurs most commonly in kids under three, and many eventually grow out of it.

Casein may also potentially cause problems if it is not broken down completely prior to its absorption in the bloodstream. In a normal, healthy digestive system, casein is broken down completely into its constituent amino acids before it is absorbed into the circulation. If there are defects in the lining of our intestinal wall (a.k.a., our leaky gut), however, casein may pass into the circulation whole. Once in the circulation, it could conceivably lead to consequences similar to that of gluten—systemic inflammation and a heightened risk of autoimmune illness. However, casein has a couple things going for it that gluten does not.

One is that while the casein in nonhuman milk isn't exactly the same as human casein, it is nonetheless closely related, as it is a protein made by fellow mammals. Gluten, on the other hand, is a plant storage protein, and not close in structure or function to anything we make in our own bodies. As such, gluten is much more likely to be recognized as a foreign substance if it enters the bloodstream. Additionally, in order for milk casein to enter into the circulation in the first place it must sneak through a defect in a leaky gut. As we've already discussed, leaky guts are typically a consequence of eating plant lectins, including those found in wheat. If we're avoiding the foods that lead to a leaky gut to begin with, then we're not providing a way for casein protein to enter the circulation intact. With an intact gut lining, the potential problems from casein become a nonissue.

Some have raised concern about a possible association between dairy consumption and cancer. A handful of observational epidemiological studies have found that, in certain populations, those individuals who had cancer had consumed more dairy than those who didn't (Fairfield et al. 2004; Larsson, Bergkuist, and Wolk 2004). Other population studies have not demonstrated this association (Moorman and Terry 2004), however, and in fact some have shown that consumption of high-fat dairy has a *protective* role against cancer (Cho et al. 2004; Larsson, Bergkuist, and Wolk 2005). One of the components of dairy fat, conjugated linoleic acid, has been shown to *suppress* the growth of cancer cells in tissue culture (Miller et al. 2003; O'Shea et al. 2000), an effect that may explain this finding. Taken together, these findings suggest that eating dairy, provided it hasn't had the fat removed (i.e., no low- or nonfat products), can reduce your risk of certain forms of cancer.

Dairy: The Verdict

Given the totality of the evidence, unless you are lactose intolerant or casein allergic, there are no compelling reasons to avoid dairy, especially if you've eliminated the other components in your diet that compromise the walls of your digestive tract. Just avoid nonfat and low-fat products, as these are just milk sugar and protein with all the potentially cancer-fighting good fat removed.

THE FINAL SUMMATION

Sugar, gluten grains, and omega-6 fatty acids: together, these three dietary elements have a clear and highly plausible link to the diseases of civilization. None of these was a meaningful part of the human diet prior to agriculture, and each has clearly established biological mechanisms by which it contributes to the diseases of civilization:

	CEREAL GRAINS	SUGAR/ FRUCTOSE	OMEGA-6 FATTY ACIDS
OBESITY	Increase in circulating insulin levels and insulin-driven fat accumulation due to carbohydrate content; concomitant suppression of fat release from the adipose tissue.	Major factor in the development of insulin resistance in the liver, a critical step in the path toward obesity and diabetes. Interferes with mechanisms for appetite regulation.	Distorted ratio of n-6 to n-3 fatty acids leads to systemic inflammation, which has been directly linked to the development of insulin resistance, obesity, and the "metabolic syndrome."
DIABETES	Continual increase in demand for insulin secretion from pancreas to clear glucose causes pancreatic burnout. Chronic systemic inflammation secondary to reaction to foreign dietary proteins contributes to peripheral insulin resistance.	Fructose-induced fatty liver disease directly linked to insulin resistance, subsequent pancreatic "burnout," and full-blown insulin-dependent diabetes.	Heightened systemic inflammation promotes the development of insulin resistance and diabetes.
CANCER	Chronic increase in circulating insulin fuels growth of cancer cells.	Fructose-induced insulin resistance leads to increasingly elevated levels of insulin, fueling growth of cancer cells.	Distorted n-6 to n-3 ratio shown to promote tumor cell proliferation in multiple forms of cancer.

ATHERO-SCLEROSIS / HARDENING OF THE ARTERIES (Heart disease, stroke, etc.)	Foreign proteins from grains absorbed into circulation elicit widespread inflammation, including inside the blood vessel walls, which lead to plaque buildup.	High amounts of fructose in the diet overwhelm the body's capacity to keep it out of the bloodstream and tissues, causing advanced glycated end products and eliciting an inflammatory response in the blood vessel walls. Fructose raises blood triglyceride levels, leading to the arterial plaque buildup that precedes heart attack and stroke.	Pro-inflammatory effects of distorted n-6 to n-3 ratio lead to widespread inflammation, including inside the blood vessel walls, leading to plaque buildup. Excess PUFA, which is highly reactive, causes LDL oxidation, leading to damage to the blood vessel walls.
AUTOIMMUNE ILLNESS	Foreign proteins from grains absorbed whole into circulation, leading to production of antibodies that cross-react with bodily tissues.		Heightened state of inflammation associated with autoimmune illness from a distorted 6:3 ratio.

It's nearly impossible to appreciate the full impact of these diseases on our lives today. They are the very things that keep our hospitals and clinics overflowing, overburdening our health care system and causing immeasurable pain and suffering. And it is simultaneously alarming and encouraging that by and large they are entirely preventable. If everyone were to change their diets accordingly today, I'd eventually be out of a job (and no, current dietary guidelines aren't a conspiratorial attempt by the health care industry to ensure a steady supply of customers).

Needless to say, I found this renewed vision of a healthy diet compelling enough to completely change my own dietary habits—and to change them in a way that directly conflicted with what I'd been taught, no less. And, as you now know, this led to a number of pleasing effects, the most significant of which was the disappearance of my migraines.

As it turns out, I'm not the only one this has happened to. After I realized the impact this way of eating was having on my own migraines, I began hearing stories from other migraineurs who had changed their diets similarly. Time and again, lifelong migraineurs like myself were celebrating the end of their migraines as I was.

Migraine: Another Disease of Civilization

My own experience with migraine and the similar experiences of so many others has led me to the inescapable conclusion that migraine, like diabetes, cancer, heart disease, and so many others, is yet another disease of civilization. In retrospect, this should come as no surprise. We didn't become the dominant species on the planet during the past 2.5 million years by having to spend every other day vomiting in a darkened cave. Migraines must now take their rightful place on the growing list of the diseases of civilization. Their inclusion among this illustrious crew means that migraines are not simply an inevitable fact of life for some but an entirely preventable consequence of our modern lifestyle and diet. Furthermore, this new conception of migraine provides us with a clear path toward migraine freedom.

Revising the Migraine Model

As we talked about in chapter 2, a migraine is a process that can be switched on inside our brains whenever our migraine risk level crosses the migraine threshold. Back before I transitioned to an ancestral diet, I crossed that threshold often. Thanks to a strong family history of migraines (unfavorable genetics) and the erratic sleep schedule that goes with taking regular hospital calls, even on a migraine-free day I was never far from the threshold. Thinking back to the migraine model presented in chapter 2, my own migraine risk level usually looked like what's shown in figure 3a.

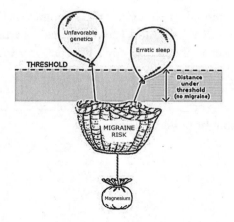

Figure 3a: Prior to changing to an ancestral diet, this was how things looked for me most days from the standpoint of the migraine model. Thanks to a strong family history and a somewhat erratic sleep schedule, my migraine risk level was never far from the threshold, despite a little risk-lowering afforded by a magnesium supplement.

As you can see, on any given day it wouldn't take much to push me beyond the threshold. A poor night's sleep, a skipped meal, or a sip of caffeinated coffee in the afternoon would easily propel me into throbbing-skull territory, represented by figure 3b.

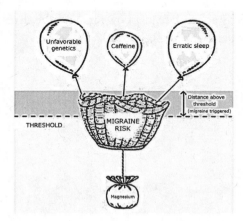

Figure 3b: Before switching to an ancestral diet, it wouldn't take more than the caffeine in a cup of coffee to lift my migraine risk level beyond the trigger threshold.

At the time, though, I thought I was doing everything I could to lower my migraine risk level, and I had accepted as a fact of life that a migraine was never more than a cup of coffee or a bite of pepperoni pizza away.

Things couldn't be more different now. With an ancestral diet, I'm able to keep my migraine risk level farther below the threshold than I ever would've thought possible (figure 3c).

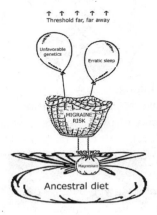

Figure 3c: Nowadays, thanks to the anchoring effect of an ancestral diet, my migraine risk level stays far away from the migraine threshold.

In fact, to fully appreciate just how far away the threshold is requires a change in our perspective (figure 3d).

MIGRAINE
- - - - - - - - - -
THRESHOLD

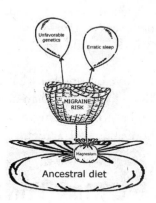

Figure 3d: On an ancestral diet, I'm so far away from the threshold that even seeing it requires a change in perspective!

And because my baseline risk level is so low, all those little things that used to send me past the threshold don't do so anymore. Because of the weight of an ancestral diet, I can sip a cup of coffee in a café while snacking on nuts and blue cheese next to an olfactorily-challenged man with overbearingly heavy cologne while my head remains blissfully pain free (figure 3e).

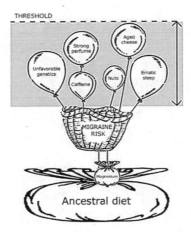

Figure 3e: The weight of an ancestral diet keeps my migraine risk level so low that even the combination of many of my old nemeses still isn't enough to lift me past the threshold.

For all these years, we've overlooked what is far and away the best weapon against migraine—far greater than any medication or supplement. When it comes to lowering our migraine risk level, nothing even compares to the weight of an ancestral diet.

How Did We Miss This?

When you stop and think about it, it's pretty remarkable that we've missed something so obvious for so long. We've long known, of course, that foods could trigger a migraine, and many migraineurs search desperately to identify anything they eat that might lead to a migraine. But if you look on any list of dietary migraine triggers, you're unlikely to find sugar, wheat, or vegetable and seed oils on it. How could that be?

If removal of these items from our diet is the most powerful weapon we have against migraines, how is it we didn't figure this out long ago?

In fact, it is precisely because these things are so prevalent in our diets that we've failed to recognize their impact on migraines (and all the diseases of civilization, for that matter) for so long. Consider for a moment the case of lung cancer. Virtually everyone knows these days that cigarette smoking is the primary cause of most cases of lung cancer. And we know this because individuals who smoke are ten to twenty times more likely to get lung cancer than those who don't. The data here is pretty unequivocal, and as a result the association between cigarettes and lung cancer has been pretty easy to identify.

But what if everybody smoked? When we look for causes of a disease, we usually start by identifying the differences (in diet, lifestyle, genetics, etc.) between those with the disease and those without. If everybody smoked, however, we'd have no way to tell that smoking had anything to do with lung cancer. Since not everyone who smokes will get cancer, there would still be folks with lung cancer and folks without it, yet there'd be no difference in smoking rates between the two groups. Instead, we'd focus on the differences that did exist between the groups. We might conclude that certain genetic mutations were the biggest risk factor, or exposures to toxins like arsenic, with no way of knowing that we were overlooking the primary culprit.

The same is true of the disease-causing agents of our modern diets—grains, sugar, and plant oils. They were ushered in by the agricultural revolution and have now become a dietary staple in virtually every modern culture. In fact, were it not for the isolated populations of humans that were never affected by the agricultural revolution, we might never have figured out their link to the diseases of civilization—including migraine.

The only missing piece in our story now is just how the modern diet leads to a migraine. We've covered how grains, sugar, and omega-6 fatty acids lead to the big diseases of civilization, but what about migraines? Just why do these dietary villains cause migraines, anyhow?

CHAPTER 4

Just Not Made for
These Times

As we learned in chapter 3, hunter-gatherer populations that exclusively eat foods that predate the agricultural revolution are immune to certain diseases, known collectively as the *diseases of civilization*. These include things like diabetes, heart disease, and cancer. We have a pretty good idea of how postagricultural foodstuffs like sugar, cereal grains, and omega-6 fatty acids lead to these diseases. But why might they lead to a migraine? In this chapter, we'll take a deep look in the brain to the place where migraines begin, a place that you'll discover is especially vulnerable to the changes wrought by our modern lifestyle and diet.

ESTABLISHING ORDER OUT OF CHAOS

Deep within the brain sits a small, almond-size structure known as the *hypothalamus*, its modest footprint belying the enormous responsibility it carries. Its function: to be the master controller of *homeostasis*, or the maintenance of stable internal bodily conditions in the midst of an ever-changing external environment.

At any given moment, an incomprehensible number of chemical reactions are occurring inside our bodies, each one critical to our health and survival. Yet, in order for these reactions to unfold properly, the conditions inside of our bodies—temperature, acid/base balance (pH), mineral concentrations, blood flow, and energy availability must be maintained within a critically narrow range. Even relatively minor disturbances in our internal state—an increase in body temperature by a few degrees or a small drop in pH—can throw the body into internal chaos. When all those chemical reactions that constitute a working human being break down, the result is dysfunction or death. So while our external environment may change dramatically throughout the course of the day, our internal environment must remain extremely stable. And it is the hypothalamus's job to ensure that it does. Without a functioning hypothalamus to maintain this stability, we die.

The Well-Connected Hypothalamus

So just how does the tiny hypothalamus accomplish such a monstrous feat? By being very well connected. The hypothalamus may be small, but it knows how to network. It receives information via nerve impulses and signaling molecules from just about every part of the body—information that provides moment-to-moment data about our internal state. It is then able to influence our internal state in a number of ways. Through its position as central commander of the endocrine system, it directs the secretion of hormones from the body's various endocrine glands (thyroid, adrenals, gonads, etc.). As chief conductor of the autonomic nervous system, it controls those vital nervous system functions that occur "automatically," beneath our conscious awareness—breathing, digestion, heart rate, sweating, salivation, and so on. Last, thanks to its widespread connections throughout the brain, it can alter our behavior in ways that promote homeostasis by generating feelings like hunger, thirst, alertness, and fatigue.

A few examples of the hypothalamus in action will help.

Temperature Regulation: When we're out in the summer heat for a while and our body temperature starts to rise, the hypothalamus, triggered by temperature receptors that detect a rise in body temperature, sends nerve impulses to the blood vessels in the skin, causing them to dilate (in other words, the skin turns red). Heat is then released from the blood across the skin. It sends signals to the sweat glands, causing the release of sweat on the skin, the evaporation of which also cools the skin's surface. Via hormone signals to the adrenal and thyroid glands, it reduces our metabolic rate and consequently our body temperature. And, through its connections to emotional centers in the brain, it makes us feel hot and unpleasant, directing us to seek out a cooler spot in the shade.

On the other hand, when we get cold, the hypothalamus directs the blood vessels in the skin to constrict, redirecting blood flow to the body's core so that heat is retained. Nerve impulses sent to the skeletal muscles make them fire rapidly, causing us to shiver and raise our body heat. Tiny muscles under our skin are activated as well, making the hairs on our skin stand up to give us "goose bumps." Back when we were furrier creatures, this helped to trap a layer of insulating air next to our skin to help retain body heat. Nowadays, it serves as a reminder of our evolutionary predecessors.

Fluid Balance: When the amount of water inside the body goes down (dehydration), receptors in the hypothalamus detect the resultant rise in blood salt concentration. The pituitary gland, under orders from the hypothalamus, releases vasopressin, a hormone that acts on the kidneys to promote water retention, giving rise to a more concentrated urine. Vasopressin also causes constriction of the blood vessels, which counteracts the blood-pressure–lowering effect of dehydration. To influence our behavior, neural impulses from the hypothalamus result in the feeling of thirst, propelling us to secure a drink of water.

Blood Glucose: When blood sugar levels drop quickly or to low levels, hypothalamic glucose detectors note the change. Once the drop is detected, the hypothalamus directs the pituitary to release ACTH (adrenocorticotropic hormone), a hormone that then stimulates the release of glucocorticoids from the adrenal glands. Together, these hormones bring blood sugar back up by, among other things, stimulating the production of glucose in the liver and suppressing glucose uptake in the tissues. In an effort to conserve energy until glucose levels are restored, the hypothalamus reduces our metabolic rate. The hypothalamus also makes us feel hungry so that we'll find some food to bring those glucose levels back up!

Circadian Rhythms: The hypothalamus is the principal regulator of our *circadian rhythms*, the biological processes that occur on a twenty-four-hour cycle. The most well known of these is our pattern of wakefulness and sleep. Naturally, these cycles developed in response to the rise and fall of the sun, and it is sunlight that the hypothalamus uses to set and regulate its twenty-four-hour clock. Light-sensing nerves in the back of the eye (retina) project directly to the hypothalamus, allowing it to precisely calibrate the clock to the time of day in order to regulate when we should be alert and awake, and when we should sleep.

Stress Response: When there's a threat to our survival or well-being, be it real or imagined, the hypothalamus engages our fight-or-flight reaction, activating the sympathetic nervous system and sending out a surge of adrenaline hormones. In response, the heart pumps harder and faster to supply more blood to the brain and muscles, the pupils dilate to let in more light, the lungs expand to let in more oxygen, blood flow is directed away from the internal organs and toward the skeletal muscles where oxygen is most needed, and the liver releases stored glucose into the bloodstream to ensure that those muscles have plenty of fuel. Like it does in response to hypoglycemia, the hypothalamus stimulates the release of cortisol and epinephrine to help ensure that enough glucose will be available if the threat lasts for more than a few minutes.

So, with these examples in mind, let's consider some factors that might tax the capabilities of the hypothalamus:

- Disruption in sleep/wake cycle (due to erratic sleep patterns, stimulants, or depressant drugs)

- Dehydration

- Overheating

- Stress

- Large fluctuations in blood sugar

Sound familiar?

If so, you're not alone. It's no surprise, given what we know about migraines and what you now know about the hypothalamus, that the hypothalamus has become a primary suspect in the hunt for the neural origins of migraine. Many of the most potent migraine triggers just so happen to fall under the domain of the hypothalamus, strong evidence supporting a central role in migraine initiation. Beyond this provocative observation, several other pieces of indirect evidence also support a tight link between a migraine and the hypothalamus.

Exhibit A: Periodicity

A migraine clearly follows a periodic pattern in many migraineurs, a feature that implicates the hypothalamus, given its primary role in the regulation of biological cycles. Some people experience their migraines predictably at a specific time of year or season, some at particular times of the month, and others at particular times of day.

Periodicity is almost a universal feature of cluster headaches, a close cousin of migraines that, like migraines, involves activation of the trigemino-vascular system. Attacks of cluster headaches often recur at very specific times of year. Once an attack begins, the headaches themselves typically recur at precisely the same time of day (often very early in the morning). For these reasons, cluster headaches are widely thought of as a disorder of the hypothalamus, given its role in regulating our day/night cycle.

The notion that cluster headaches are a disorder of the hypothalamus has led researchers to attempt an experimental treatment in which a small stimulating electrode is surgically implanted into the hypothalamus. Early results indicate that they've found the right target. In one study (May et al. 2006), electrode stimulation in the hypothalamus resulted in complete resolution of cluster headaches in eight of ten subjects. Interestingly, stimulation in the hypothalamus did not affect pain-sensing regions of the brain, leading researchers to conclude that the effect on headache remission was at a more fundamental level.

Exhibit B: Sexual Dimorphism

Clear differences exist between the sexes when it comes to migraines. In most analyses, the rate of migraine headaches is roughly three times greater in women than men. This disparity offers another clue in our search for the origins of migraine, beckoning us to look to areas of the brain that are also different between men and women, or that are, in scientific terms, "sexually dimorphic." Once again, the hypothalamus turns up as a prime suspect. While most brain regions vary little between the sexes, the hypothalamus is a conspicuous exception. Within the hypothalamus are multiple nuclei, clusters of cells that are grouped according to functional similarities. Several of these nuclei differ considerably between men and women in their size, connectivity, and chemical sensitivity.

Along these same lines, the tendency for migraines to worsen during times of major hormonal changes also argues for hypothalamic involvement. As mentioned previously, migraines often worsen considerably during the first trimester of pregnancy, a time of massive hormonal changes in the female body. And the association between the menstrual cycle and migraines has long been recognized, so much so that it has spawned its own diagnostic category. Specifically, the fall in estrogen levels that precedes menses correlates most strongly with the onset of migraine headaches—an observation that naturally led to speculation that estrogen replacement could cure menstrual migraines. Yet these trials have not been successful, a fact that suggests that the fundamental problem, while correlated in time with the drop in estrogen release from the ovaries, lies elsewhere. Once again, the hypothalamus rears its head.

Exhibit C: The Prodrome

In chapter 1, we discovered that for many, migraines begin with a prodromal phase, a period lasting up to forty-eight hours when a variety of premonitory symptoms might be experienced. These include things like hunger, food cravings, thirst, fatigue, fluid retention, and heat intolerance. All of these are signs of disordered homeostatic regulation, which manifests in hunger despite adequate energy stores and thirst despite adequate body water, among other signs. In other words, the earliest signs of migraine are those of a malfunctioning hypothalamus.

All of this circumstantial evidence hasn't gone unnoticed by the migraine research community, and in recent years, the case against the hypothalamus has been strengthened further. In particular, our ability to look at the migraine brain in real time with functional brain imaging can show us which parts of the brain are active during a migraine, and when. And, indeed, when the brain of a migraineur is imaged early in the course of a migraine, the hypothalamus is teeming with activity (Denuelle et al. 2007).

Needless to say, the case against the hypothalamus is strong. Clearly it plays a major role in migraines, and there is convincing evidence that it is the place where it all begins. The best available evidence indicates that the migraine switch we discussed in chapter 2 is housed inside of it.

A FISH OUT OF WATER

In the previous chapter we discussed the idea of migraine as a disease of civilization, an affliction that only exists among humans in the postagricultural era. As a species, we've spent 2.5 million years living as hunter-gatherers, and as a result our bodies, and our brains, are highly adapted to this way of life. Yet the conditions we find ourselves in these days bear little resemblance to those of our prehistoric ancestors, especially when we consider the technological advances that have occurred in the past couple of centuries. In many facets of life, our body, including the hypothalamus, is faced with a *mismatch* between its current conditions and the conditions it expects. And if the hypothalamus is the part of the brain where migraine begins, where the switch is located, then understanding the differences between these two ways of life from its point of view holds the key to understanding why migraines occur. Perhaps more importantly, it holds the key to stopping them.

Mismatch 1: Sleep/Wake Cycle

In our prehistoric days, we rose when the sun came up and slept when it went down. As discussed, the hypothalamic clock is set by the comings and goings of the sun. Nowadays, thanks largely to the invention of the incandescent bulb, we no longer require the sun to light the world around us. We're free to wake up and go to sleep when we please—dawn and dusk have been relegated to spectator events rather than the master regulators of our biological clock that they once were.

Mismatch 2: Stress!

Before the advent of civilization, we spent our lives in small groups, living alongside our immediate and extended families for much of our days. The rest of our tribe also likely consisted of people we knew well. These were people we cared for and who cared for us. We are social creatures, and these closely knit societies both nourished our spirits and provided us with a rich support structure we could draw upon during times of need. Challenges were seldom faced alone. We depended on the people around us, and they on us.

These days, though we may live in places where the population density is much higher, our connections to those around us are, in many cases, far more tenuous and superficial. Many of us live far away from our immediate families. Many of us have never even met much of our extended family. For many, our neighbors are just the people we wave hello to from our driver's seat on the way into the garage. We don't depend on them, and they don't depend on us.

This erosion of our social support structure has no doubt had an impact, most notably on our mental health, in particular our capacity to handle stress. Among my own patients, complaints about stress are nearly universal. In medical school we were told that roughly half or more of our patient visits would stem from psychological issues, a claim I was at the time quite skeptical of. An audit of my patient charts, however, reveals it to be true. To our bodies, this means that more and more of us are spending more and more of our time with our body's stress response activated—a response coordinated by the hypothalamus.

That's not to say that stress didn't exist among our hunter-gatherer ancestors. It most certainly did. The very fact that we have such a complex and highly organized biological response to stress tells us that it did, and it tells us that our ability to respond appropriately to stress has been key to human survival for a long time. Yet our ancestors' was likely a very different kind of stress.

When our precivilized ancestors faced a threat, it was in the form of a very tangible and self-limited challenge to survival, such as an encounter with a wild animal, an approaching storm, or a physical injury. The threat was very real, and the activation of our stress response adaptive. These days, the nature of the stress that permeates day-to-day life is often of a very different sort—it is intangible and open ended. It's a type of stress generated by thought alone—anxiety about money, relationships, job performance, and so on. As such, it has no defined end. In this case, the activation of our stress response, designed to respond to the challenges a hunter-gatherer might face, is *maladaptive*. Not only does it interfere with our ability to deal with the very things we're worried about, but it also wreaks continual havoc on our bodies. Stress hormones that previously would've been released in short bursts every once in a while instead float around in the bloodstream regularly. And, while the type of stress we face these days is very different *in kind*, to the body (and to the hypothalamus) it seems just the same. To our hypothalamus, it's as if we live in a world where there's a wild boar on every corner, ready to pounce.

Mismatch 3: Energy Consumption

And last, let's not forget the stuff we eat. From the perspective of the hypothalamus, perhaps nothing has changed more than the wild and unpredictable swings in blood glucose brought about by our shift to an agriculturally-based and increasingly processed diet. From the hypothalamus's point of view, our nearly forty-fold increase in sugar consumption represents arguably the greatest departure from our ancestral environment. And maintaining energy homeostasis in such an unfamiliar milieu may well be its single greatest challenge.

FAT-ADAPTED METABOLISM: LEAVING THE BLOOD SUGAR ROLLER COASTER

To operate, the human body requires a continual source of energy. Even while we sleep, basic functions must continue to run, or else we don't stay alive for very long. When it comes to where we humans can derive that energy, we're actually quite flexible, relatively speaking. To power the zillions of chemical reactions taking place inside our bodies, we can burn either glucose or fat (or, more specifically, fatty acids). Generally speaking, we acquire that glucose and fat from one of two places:

- The food we eat

- Stored forms of fat and glucose inside our bodies

Fat-Burning Hunter-Gatherers

When our body is running primarily on fatty acids, our metabolism is primarily fat centered, or *adipocentric*. When it is running primarily on sugar, our metabolism is primarily glucose centered, or *glucocentric*. To the body, these two metabolic states are quite different, utilizing a unique set of metabolic machinery that requires the upregulation and expression of differing sets of genes. Switching from one mode of operation to another is a process that takes time. A complete transition from glucocentric to adipocentric metabolism can take up to a few weeks to occur.

In our hunter-gatherer days, access to dietary glucose was quite limited. Most of the energy we obtained from food was either from fat, which could be burned directly for energy, or to a lesser extent from protein, which can be converted inside the body to glucose. During times of food abundance, most of our energy needs were met by burning dietary fat. In those days, we also faced periods when food was scarce, forcing us to rely on our body's energy stores. Our capacity to store energy as glucose is very limited—we don't store enough to even meet our energy needs for one day. Our capacity to store energy as fat, on the other hand, is substantial. A 140-pound woman with a healthy body fat of 20 percent (or 12,700 grams of fat) has enough stored energy in her adipose tissue to meet energy needs for roughly two months. For a modern-day human stuck in glucocentric metabolism, however, this rich fuel source isn't so easy to get to. Our precivilized, adipocentric ancestors, on the other hand, could tap in to their stored fat easily, so that in times of food shortages they could still meet their energy needs and continue to thrive.

So for two million years, regardless of whether food was plentiful or scarce, our bodies ran mainly on fat. It has been our preferred fuel source for almost the entirety of human evolution.

Sugar-Burning Modern Man

These days, access to dietary sugars is essentially unlimited. Carbohydrates, particularly of the refined variety, are ubiquitous and cheap. Furthermore, we've been told by the powers that be that they should be our primary food source, occupying pole position at the base of the food pyramid. Not surprisingly, most folks consume the bulk of their energy from dietary sugars, resulting in a metabolism that is primarily glucocentric. One of the consequences of always being in glucocentric-sugar-burning mode is that it limits our ability to tap in to the stored energy in our fat tissue. As stated, the metabolic machinery required to access these fat stores readily is suppressed, and bringing it back up takes time.

Here's how this plays out day to day: After a carbohydrate-heavy meal, there's a large spike in blood sugar. In response, the pancreas releases insulin, which drives glucose into the tissues. The cells inside those tissues then use that glucose to meet their energy needs for the next several hours. Eventually, blood glucose starts to fall. For an efficient fat-burning human (our ancestors included), this doesn't create a problem. They can just switch easily to burning their stored fat. For those dependent on sugar, however, it creates an energy crisis—an energy crisis sensed by the hypothalamus. The result: ravenous hunger and massive crankiness. That ravenous hunger persists until the next hit of sugar, and the cycle begins anew. This is the energy roller coaster of a carbohydrate-heavy, glucocentric diet. And, to the hypothalamus, it's as if we face the threat of starvation every day.

Glucocentric metabolism is the norm nowadays, thanks to our carbohydrate-rich diets. As such, most folks consider the subsequent large fluctuations in energy levels, appetite, and mood that occur throughout the course of the day to be unavoidable facts of life. Yet, it isn't. Not only is it an unnecessarily unpleasant way to live, it also raises the level of difficulty for the hypothalamus to maintain energy constancy. When we've adapted to using fat as our primary fuel source, we experience just the opposite—minimal fluctuations in energy levels, appetite, and mood. If you've ever wondered why low-carbohydrate diets work so well and are so popular, this is it. For weight loss, low-carb diets consistently outperform traditional calorie-restricted (calorie-counting) diets in controlled studies (Gardner et al. 2007; Brehm et al. 2003; Samaha et al. 2003; Volek et al. 2004) in large part because compliance is so much better. People on low-carb diets report far less hunger, despite typically consuming fewer calories than their starving calorie-counting comrades. Thanks to their newfound ability to access their fat stores, they've said good-bye to the glucocentric energy roller coaster. Burning those fat stores for energy also means they're losing weight—another cause for celebration.

From the vantage point of the hypothalamus, there is perhaps no greater contrast between the modern and hunter-gatherer lifestyle than our diet and the resultant instability in energy availability. And if the hypothalamus is the birthplace of migraine, it's not surprising then that reverting back to the diet of our ancestors is our greatest weapon against it.

INSIGHTS FROM THE KETOGENIC DIET

To neurologists, there are many similarities between migraines and seizures. Both are episodic. Both reflect temporary changes in brain states, often with localized neurochemical disturbances. Both are provoked by many of the same things: stress, erratic sleep cycles, stimulants, and sedatives. Both are suppressed to some extent by medications that calm "overactive" brain cells.

Since the 1920s, the *ketogenic diet* has been a powerful tool in treating children who have intractable seizures—seizures that persist, in many cases occurring daily, in spite of all attempts to control them with medications. The ketogenic diet is a high-fat, low-carbohydrate diet. As mentioned above, reducing the amount of dietary carbohydrates in the diet shifts our metabolism from sugar-centered to fat-centered. Another consequence of a low-carbohydrate diet is that it also increases the production of *ketone bodies*, or *ketones*, by the liver. If dietary carbohydrates are dropped low enough—under 50 grams per day (sometimes less)—ketone bodies start appearing in the urine, and the body is said to be in a state of *ketosis*. Achieving ketosis is the goal of the ketogenic diet. Multiple variations of the ketogenic diet exist, but they all share this common objective.

So what is it about a high-fat, low-carbohydrate ketogenic diet that makes it so effective at preventing seizures? Well, the truth is that we still don't know for sure, as epilepsy researchers have only recently begun to try to answer this question. One potential explanation is the effect that ketosis has on the brain's energy utilization. When we're in sugar-burning mode, the brain runs almost exclusively on glucose. The brain can't burn fatty acids because they cannot cross the blood-brain barrier. Ketone bodies, on the other hand, cross this barrier easily. And the brain can burn ketones directly for energy. In a ketogenic diet, up to three-quarters of the brain's energy needs are met by ketones (the remainder by glucose)—a drastic change from the typical modern diet. This shift itself from the utilization of glucose to the utilization of ketones for energy may be responsible for the reduction in seizures (Gasior, Rogawski, and Hartman 2006). Seizures, like migraines, may not propagate well using ketones for fuel. Or, to put it another way, seizures, like migraines, may propagate *really well* when the brain is running purely on glucose.

Another intriguing finding from this line of research is that ketones may prevent cellular injury. Experiments have shown that ketone bodies protect brain cells from oxidative damage and destruction (Maalouf, Rho, and Mattson 2009). This type of damage, perpetrated by free radicals, is thought to be a major player in many degenerative diseases of the brain, including Alzheimer's, Parkinson's, and Lou Gehrig's disease (ALS) (Srikanth et al. 2011; Münch et al. 1998; Barber and Shaw 2010). These findings have opened up a tantalizing line of research, as ketogenic diets are now being investigated as a potential treatment for these disorders.

It is also possible that the ketone bodies themselves are directly responsible for the seizure reduction. Some studies (Gasior, Rogawski, and Hartman 2006) have shown that ketones can inhibit brain signaling, suppressing the function of the hyperactive brain cells that spark seizures.

So you might wonder, naturally, if the ketogenic diet is so effective at reducing seizures in children—typically succeeding when prescription medications have failed—why is it only used as a last resort? Sadly, it has almost everything to do with our irrational and unfounded fear of fat. Specifically, it stems from the fear that a high-fat diet will "clog the arteries" and lead to heart disease and other vascular problems. And so, the ketogenic diet has been considered "dangerous" because of concerns over possible long-term cardiovascular complications. Furthermore, even though many have suspected that the ketogenic diet would also be effective at preventing migraines, it has not been formally studied out of similar concerns, save for a few case reports describing complete resolution of migraine headaches with a ketogenic diet (Strahlman 2006; Urbizu et al. 2010; Schnabel 1928).

Now, from what we've covered in the last chapter, we know that this purported connection between fat and heart disease is entirely without merit. Additionally, we also now know that the ketogenic diet itself has no long-term side effects, including no adverse effects on the cardiovascular system, thanks to a 2010 study published by Dr. Amisha Patel and colleagues at Johns Hopkins involving 101 patients who had been on a ketogenic diet long term. On the contrary, the ketogenic diet has been shown (in obese patients, no less) to raise HDL cholesterol, lower serum triglyceride levels, and lower fasting blood sugar—all of which confer a marked *reduction* in the risk of heart disease (Westman et al. 2008; Yancy et al. 2004). Ironically, the ketogenic diet isn't just a powerful weapon against seizures; it's even a powerful weapon *against* heart disease! That it has yet to become a first-line therapy for children with epilepsy illustrates just how firmly entrenched our fear of fat has become, as irrational as it is. It's the myth that won't die, and we're paying the price with our health.

INFLAMMATION AND THE HYPOTHALAMUS

As discussed in the last chapter, our modern diet, through a variety of mechanisms, results in widespread systemic inflammation— inflammation that is at the heart of so many diseases of civilization. It has become increasingly clear in recent years that the hypothalamus is not spared from the diet-induced inflammatory process. In the short term, like in an acute viral infection, a rise in inflammatory substances in the hypothalamus may trigger the fever, lethargy, and loss of appetite that is part of our natural adaptive response to infection. Longer-term diet-induced inflammation, however, disrupts the hypothalamus's normal operation. We're currently in the midst of an epidemic of metabolic syndrome, composed of the triad of obesity, insulin resistance, and hypertension. The fact that these three conditions so commonly emerge together has naturally led to speculation that there's a common fundamental cause. Each of these conditions represents a breakdown in homeostatic regulation (body fat, blood sugar, and blood pressure), leading researchers to look to the hypothalamus as the possible source of these problems. Indeed, in animal studies, diet-induced inflammation of the hypothalamus results in the development of metabolic syndrome, supporting the notion that hypothalamic inflammation and resultant dysfunction is at the heart of this epidemic (Cai and Liu 2012).

So, in other words, not only does the modern world (and the modern diet) pose an unprecedented and unfamiliar challenge to the homeostatic capacity of the hypothalamus, but diet-induced inflammation also directly compromises its ability to respond to that challenge. We've not only asked the hypothalamus to perform a job it wasn't designed for, we've asked it to do so with one hand tied behind its back!

GUIDE TO A HAPPY HYPOTHALAMUS

To recap, we've learned in this chapter that the hypothalamus is, at the very least, an integral part of the migraine process, and quite likely the place where it all begins.

The hypothalamus, being the principal regulator of homeostasis, faces an enormous challenge: namely, to maintain stable internal body conditions in the modern world. It's a world far different than the one it was designed for through millions of years of adaptation. It's as if it has woken up one day to find itself in an unfamiliar land and been asked to perform a job that it has never prepared for. It struggles mightily to rise to the challenge, and the fact that it performs as well as it does is testament to the remarkable adaptability of the human body and brain. But the cost of that struggle, for many, is migraines.

Yet the upside of this newfound perspective on migraines is that it gives us a clear guiding principle to achieve migraine freedom. To prevent migraines, our directive is simple: re-create, as best we can, the conditions that the hypothalamus was designed for.

Directive 1: Maintain a Stable Sleep/Wake Cycle

In an ideal world, this would mean waking when the sun rises and going to sleep when it falls. Still, entraining our day and night patterns as closely as possible to the rhythms of the sun is a worthy goal. Even if we can't attain this ideal, we can at least work toward a consistent day and night cycle. This means waking and sleeping at roughly the same time each day, and giving ourselves enough time to sleep. Our hypothalamus, as the part of the brain that makes us feel awake or sleepy, can still be a valuable ally in helping us to maintain this consistency, provided we help it do so by providing it the input it needs. This includes pursuing every opportunity to take in natural light during the course of the day. And it means limiting our exposure to artificial light sources after the sun has set. Blue light is the worst offender when it comes to disrupting our hypothalamic clock, while light in the yellow range of the visible spectrum makes less of an impact.

Unfortunately, the light of our computer screens, smartphones, and flat-screen televisions is heavy in the blue spectrum (on the upside, exposing yourself to these sources of light during the day actually helps entrain your clock). And, if turning them off entirely after the sun has set isn't a viable option, there are ways to minimize their impact. The program f.lux, which you can install on your computer, will automatically reduce the amount of blue light emitted by your computer in the evening. Additionally, if you are having difficulty maintaining a consistent sleep schedule, taking a short course of melatonin, a hormone that is naturally secreted by the pineal gland under the direction of the hypothalamus to promote sleep, can help entrain the sleep/wake cycle.

A typical regimen is 5 milligrams (available over the counter) taken an hour before bedtime for four weeks.

Directive 2: Reduce Stress

Here of course I'm talking primarily about psychological stress—the nagging worry and anxiety that seem to permeate our existence these days. As mentioned, one of the things we benefited most from emotionally in our hunter-gatherer days was an extensive support structure that included both our immediate and extended family. Communal activities were the norm. Though we may not live with or near family, we can still work to create our own network of support, as it is one of the most important determinants of our psychological well-being, fortifying us in times of stress. Furthermore, finding a reliable method for relieving stress when it does occur, and incorporating that method into your daily routine, is a must.

Directive 3: Move Your Body

We didn't always spend so much of our time sitting in chairs or sofas, glued to computers or television sets. Before the advent of agriculture and modern conveniences, there were animals to be hunted, plants to be gathered, and fires to be tended. Sure, our ancestors still made time for rest and relaxation, but physical activity during the day was the norm. This doesn't mean you need to wander around all day in a loincloth hunting for berries, but it does mean incorporating some kind of physical activity into your daily routine. Even something as simple as a brisk walk for thirty minutes a day confers broad health benefits. And, as discussed earlier, a program of regular exercise has been shown to be as effective at preventing migraines as the best available prescription medications (Varkey et al. 2011).

Directive 4: Eat Like Your Ancestors

To the hypothalamus, nothing has changed more than the way we eat. Because of agriculture and modern methods of food production, more than half of our calories now comes from foods our hunter-gatherer ancestors never ate. The result is widespread inflammation, chronic disease, and an internal metabolic environment very different from the one the hypothalamus was designed to manage. Restoring our internal metabolic environment to that of our ancestors is the single most important thing we can do to maximize our capacity for long-term health and vitality. It is also the single biggest thing we can do to unburden our overworked and inflamed hypothalami so that we may live our lives free of migraines.

CHAPTER 5

The Miracle "Diet"

So you've finally arrived. You're now an expert in migraine physiology and well versed in all of the conventional options for migraine treatment. You also now understand nutrition and disease in an entirely new light, and you appreciate the importance of an ancestral diet in maintaining health and preventing migraines. All that's left is for you to translate that knowledge into action and begin your own journey toward a healthier, migraine-free future. It's time now for the rubber to meet the road.

"DIET": A CLARIFICATION

First things first—this isn't really a "diet." At least not in the way many people think of the word. To most people these days, "diet" means a temporary departure from the things you usually eat—a time-limited approach to weight loss or some other goal. Oftentimes when I pose the question "What's your diet like?" I'm met with the response "Oh, I'm not on a diet."

But this isn't a diet in that sense—it's merely a way of eating for optimal health and an end to migraines. This eating plan is presented as six primary directives that, when followed, eliminate the items in the modern diet that were introduced by the agricultural and industrial revolution *and* that are most closely linked to the diseases of civilization. It is up to you to decide how to implement the directives, be it step by step or all at once. To some, doing it all at once may seem too daunting. To others, an all-or-nothing approach works best. I've had patients who've been equally successful using either method, and you probably know which camp you fall into.

Directive 1: Eliminate Foods with Flour (Wheat, Barley, and Rye) and Added Sugar

This is the step most people find the most intimidating. It is also the one that will impact your health and migraines the most, which is why I have listed it first. If you do nothing else but eliminate sugar and flour from your diet, you will have made an enormous change for the better.

I understand the intimidation, though. I was there once myself. *A life without sandwiches?! No buttered bread before meals? What on earth will I eat?!*

Flour and sugar (cane sugar, high-fructose corn syrup, etc.) are cheap and convenient sources of calories. And, thanks in no small part to the mainstream health community's willingness to ignore, dismiss, or downplay their potential harms, they have become staples of the standard Western diet. Yet, despite the fact that flour and sugar compose the major caloric source for most folks these days (Lindeberg 2010), in reality they represent only a tiny blip in the spectrum of available foods. Rest assured, there's plenty still left to eat without them in your diet—if our human ancestors were able to get along for 2.5 million years without flour and sugar (in a world without supermarkets, no less!), certainly we can as well. For many, successful implementation of this step is primarily a matter of forming new habits. And old habits die hard, for sure. Though the first few weeks may require some thoughtful planning and concerted effort, soon enough you'll find eating this way to be second nature. Once this happens, you may look back and wonder why giving up flour and sugar ever seemed like such a big deal.

Though the term "flour" is most often used synonymously with "wheat flour" (as in this discussion), it is worth pointing out that it is the flour from the gluten grains that you should avoid, which include not only wheat but also barley and rye. These days, thanks to the ever-expanding awareness of gluten sensitivity and intolerance, you may find more and more non-gluten grain flours (rice, sorghum, buckwheat) on grocery store shelves. While these alternatives are also a dense source of dietary carbohydrate, they do not possess the same dangers as the gluten-grain flours, and as such are fine to use in moderation.

Beyond its effect on migraine reduction, let's review what else you stand to gain by eliminating added sugar and flour from your diet:

- Removal of the damaging effects of excess dietary fructose, most notably of elevated triglycerides, fatty liver disease and scarring, insulin resistance, and full-blown metabolic syndrome (diabetes, high blood pressure, and obesity)

- Upregulation of the enzymatic machinery used to burn stored fatty acids, resulting in loss of excess body fat and stable blood sugar and energy levels

- Restoration of the integrity of the intestinal lining through the elimination of wheat lectin and gluten, lowering systemic inflammation and eliminating the risk of gluten-induced autoimmune illness

- Increase in nutrient absorption through reduced intake of nutrient-binding phytic acid and replacement of nutrient-rich foods for nutrient-poor wheat flour and sugar

Remember, too, that it is estimated that 30 percent or more of the population is gluten sensitive. This means you have a one in three chance of feeling a whole lot better in short order.

Directive 2: Eliminate Processed Foods (Or Only Eat Whole Foods)

In general, when deciding whether to consume a particular food, first ask yourself if it is something you could either hunt and kill or grow in a garden. Processed foods, as their name implies, do not fulfill this criteria—they require some sort of "processing" to turn them into a food product. With rare exception, if it comes in a colorful box and can spend long periods of time in your pantry without spoiling, it probably doesn't belong inside your body. Since the majority of processed foods (crackers, snack cakes, cereal, energy bars, sodas, etc.) contain added sugar, flour, or both, directive one takes care of many of the potential foods here.

Directive 3: Eat Mostly Animals and Plants

Thanks to our long evolutionary history of consuming the meat of other animals, we're well adapted to eat almost anything with legs, fins, or wings. Animals are a rich source of energy and nutrients. This includes their organ meats, which are a dense energy source and likely were a favored part of the animal for most of human history.

Most of the plant kingdom, on the other hand, is not suitable as food for humans (like cereal grains!). Since plants can't run or bite, they discourage us from eating them by making us ill when we do so. Some plants can even kill us if we ingest them. Fortunately, we have a couple of million years of accumulated cultural wisdom to draw upon (a process that likely cost more than a few prehistoric humans their lives).

Based on what we know of modern-day hunter-gatherer societies, our ancestors valued most those plants that were packed with energy. This makes perfect sense, as it would be wasteful, and potentially deadly, to spend your whole day gathering leafy greens when they couldn't even supply your body with a few minutes of fuel. Instead they preferred to spend their valuable gathering energies collecting starchy tubers and root vegetables—plants that would offer them the most bang for their gathering buck. This includes things like yams, sweet potatoes, squash, turnips, jicama, beets, plantains, taro, rutabaga, potatoes, and cassava. These days, we have the luxury of an incredible array of food options. As such, we can afford to eat leafy greens or other low-energy vegetables if desired, provided we're meeting our energy needs with other items in our diet.

Directive 4: Cook with Butter, Animal Fat, Coconut Oil, Olive Oil, or Ghee (Clarified Butter)

Don't cook with canola, seed, or grain-derived oils. Vegetable and seed oils were made possible by the industrial revolution, and as such are very new additions to the human diet. They are high in unstable, oxidation-prone omega-6 fatty acids that tip the biological scale toward widespread, systemic inflammation. Butter, animal fats (including lard, tallow, and duck fat), coconut, olive oil, and ghee are all high in saturated fat. Unlike the omega-6 PUFAs that are highly reactive when in contact with oxygen, saturated fatty acids are very stable. The same properties that render them the better choice as a dietary fat source also make them great for your pantry, as their stability in the presence of oxygen means they can be stored at room temperature for long periods without going rancid. Don't forget to read labels to make sure an unhealthy oil hasn't been snuck into the food you're buying.

Directive 5: When Eating Fruit, Favor Berries of Various Sorts over the Sweeter Stuff

In general, the sweeter fruits (bananas, apples, grapes, pears) are less nutritionally dense *and* will also lead to a sharper rise in blood sugar, which, as a migraineur, is something you wish to avoid. This doesn't mean you need to give up sweet fruits, just eat them in moderation, and always in the context of a larger meal (which helps to blunt the blood sugar rise). For many, eating a sweet fruit on an empty stomach is a big migraine trigger. The same goes for concentrated fruit juices, which should be avoided.

Berries, on the other hand, *are* both nutritionally dense and lower in sugar, and as such should be the fruits you reach for first.

Directive 6: Drink Mainly Water

Unsweetened tea (or tea sweetened with stevia or Splenda) and coffee (with or without cream or natural sweetener) are also perfectly fine in moderation. Avoid alcohol for the first few weeks of the diet. Once your migraines are well under control, you can experiment with drinking it again in moderation. Wine and clear liquors are best. Beer can be problematic for some, particularly those who are gluten sensitive (though gluten-free options continue to expand). Avoid sweetened cocktails. And, regardless of what alcohol you drink, don't overdo it, or a migraine is a virtual certainty.

FINER POINTS

If you are lactose intolerant or allergic to milk proteins (casein allergy), then avoid milk, soft cheeses, and cream (butter and hard cheeses are still generally fine). If you aren't, then dairy is generally fine. Just remember to avoid low- or nonfat products—drink whole milk, eat full-fat yogurt, use cream in your coffee, and so on.

When feasible, consume animals that were raised as close to their natural setting as possible. In general, animals in factory farms live in conditions far removed from their natural setting (conditions many consider to be inhumane). In most cases, the food they're given is a far cry from what they'd eat in the wild. Just as we aim to eat a diet that is evolutionarily appropriate for our species, we want the same to be true of the animals we eat. Factory-raised animals also typically receive antibiotics to prevent infections that result from their close quarters and unnatural diets (Diez-Gonzalez et al. 1998; Snowder et al. 2006). They may be given hormones to encourage growth. Suffice it to say, then, that they differ in these ways from the animals our ancestors ate. Fortunately, the growing movement toward sustainable agriculture and humanely raised livestock continues to expand the available marketplace of foods that fulfill our criteria. Your best bet is to know the farmer you buy your food from (and even visit his or her farm if possible). Local farmers' markets, which are popping up in more and more places these days, are the best places to find these items. Otherwise, look for "grass fed" beef and "pastured" pork, chicken, and eggs when shopping for groceries for an indicator of animals raised under natural conditions (unfortunately, the "organic" label doesn't guarantee that an animal was raised humanely).

Eat when you're hungry, stop when you're satisfied. When it comes to how frequently you should eat, the primary directive is to *listen to your body*. One of the great benefits of eating an ancestral diet is that the feelings of hunger and satiety, no longer subverted by evolutionarily inappropriate foods, are now adaptive and beneficial. In other words, you can leave it to the hidden wisdom of your body to decide how often to eat. You may well find after eating this way for some time that you can go much longer between meals than you used to. This isn't surprising, as the three-meals-a-day habit is a very recent development in human history. Our ancestors likely didn't eat three squares a day, and you needn't either if it doesn't suit you. They also likely fasted for extended periods of time with minimal discomfort when food was scarce. As a species, we are designed to easily adapt to the ebb and flow of food availability, provided we're eating an evolutionarily appropriate diet. Freedom from the three-meals-a-day confinement is yet another of the perks of eating this way.

For those with more than four migraines per month, limit carbohydrates to less than 100 grams per day for at least the first two weeks. Shifting from a sugar-centric to a fat-centric metabolism is one of the primary goals of this way of eating, and this shift is determined in large part by the amount of carbohydrates in the diet. The fewer carbohydrates, the faster this shift will occur.

For those with more than ten migraines per month, limit carbohydrates to less than 50 grams per day for the first two weeks. At this level of carbohydrate consumption, there will be significant production of ketone bodies in the liver, which can be burned by the brain in place of glucose for energy, conferring additional protective benefit against migraines. As mentioned earlier, there is now speculation that ketones may also offer protection against neurodegenerative disorders like Alzheimer's and Parkinson's diseases (Stafstrom and Rho 2012).

You may crave carbohydrates and sugar initially. During the first week or two after shifting to this way of eating, your body will be going through some significant changes as it ramps up its fat-burning machinery. It takes the body about a week or two to fully adapt to this change. During this period, you may find yourself craving sugar, and a small percentage of folks may feel lethargic. This is particularly true if you were consuming a diet fairly high in sugar (sodas, packaged snack foods, etc.) beforehand. Eating fruit and using natural sweeteners occasionally can help. Once the transition is complete, the cravings will disappear, and avoiding carbs and sweets will become much easier.

Get your vitamin D. Most of us spend far more time indoors than our prehistoric ancestors. Since much of our bodily stores of vitamin D are produced in the skin after exposure to sunlight, many of us have become vitamin D deficient—I'd estimate that about four out of every five patients I test for it are below the recommended range. At the least, low vitamin D levels will result in poor bone health, raising your risk of osteoporosis and pathological fractures. However, given its influence on processes throughout the body, there is concern that we've only begun to scratch the surface in understanding the impact of insufficient vitamin D stores.

The best way to ensure that your body is replete with vitamin D is to get plenty of midday sun (without sunscreen, which blocks the ultraviolet light needed for vitamin D production). In general, about 20 to 30 minutes of midday sun for a lighter-skinned individual is an adequate amount. Darker-skinned individuals should aim for around an hour or so. If this isn't feasible for you, then supplement with 1,000 to 2,000 International Units (IUs) of vitamin D daily.

Exercise. Reduction in migraine headache frequency is just one of the many benefits of exercise. As mentioned in chapter 3, a regular program of exercise has been shown to be as effective as the leading prescription medication in preventing migraines. No need to overdo it, either—to reap the benefits, around twenty minutes of moderate-intensity exercise (50 to 70 percent of your maximum heart rate) three times a week is all you need.

Medium-Chain Fatty Acids and the Magic of Coconut Milk

As discussed, the presence of ketone bodies in the brain can offer additional protection against migraines, as they do in epilepsy. One way to generate ketone bodies is to eat a very low carbohydrate diet of under 50 grams per day. There is another path to ketone production, however, and it involves eating foods that contain *medium-chain triglycerides*, or MCTs, of which coconut is a fantastic choice. Coconut is a rich source of saturated fat, and the majority of that saturated fat is in the form of MCTs, which have some unique and special properties. The most relevant of these for migraineurs is that MCTs are converted directly into ketone bodies in the liver. This means that consumption of MCT-rich coconut will generate the migraineur-friendly ketone bodies even if you're not restricting carbohydrate intake. Both coconut oil and coconut milk are excellent ways to add these ketone-generating fats into your diet. My typical breakfast these days is a smoothie with a cup of coconut milk in it. In the next chapter, you'll learn several ways to incorporate coconut into your diet.

DIETARY MYTHS TO EXPUNGE FROM YOUR BRAIN

Successful transition to an ancestral diet for some will require significant reframing of some long-held notions about a healthy diet. By now, these presumed truths may be so intimately woven into the fabric of your neural circuitry that they resist eradication, popping up when least expected to sabotage your efforts. What's more, they are also continually reinforced by the popular media, who've yet to catch on to the fact that the low-fat movement has been an epic failure. Having shepherded many folks now through this nutritional transition, I know how easy it is for these myths to insidiously creep back into their subconscious and stifle their progress. So to fortify you against a surreptitious attack, let's tackle these one by one.

Myth: Eating fat makes you fat.

Reality: Just as eating too many bananas won't necessarily turn you into one, eating fat will also not necessarily make you fat. In general, energy is stored as fat in the adipose tissue when we consume more energy than our immediate needs require (so it is stored to be used later), regardless of whether that energy is from fat, protein, or carbohydrate. Furthermore, low-carbohydrate, higher-fat diets consistently outperform low-fat diets in head-to-head studies, even when the low-fat dieters are counting their calories (Brehm et al. 2003; Samaha et al. 2003; Volek et al. 2004). Most people eat fewer calories, or consume less energy, when eating a low-carbohydrate, high-fat meal than when eating a low-fat, high-carbohydrate one.

A high-carbohydrate diet also suppresses the enzymatic machinery required to burn fat from the adipose tissue, making it more difficult to readily access fat stores when needed—another factor that likely impedes weight loss on low-fat diets. Remember, too, that fat is stored under the direction of insulin, and insulin secretion is governed by the amount of *carbohydrates* in the bloodstream.

Myth: Animal fat leads to clogged arteries.

Reality: The idea that animal fat, particularly the saturated kind, leads to heart disease has been squarely refuted by scientific evidence (Siri-Tarino et al. 2010), yet it remains one of the most intractable modern health myths. Humans have been consuming the meat of other animals for a very long time. Among modern-day hunter-gatherer societies whose diets are very high in animal fat, heart disease and stroke are medical odditites (Trowell and Burkitt 1981; Lindeberg 2010). Our modern diet, on the other hand, is extraordinarily high in the proinflammatory omega-6 fats found in plants, thanks to the introduction of industrially processed vegetable and seed oils into our diets. In controlled studies, replacement of vegetable fat for animal fat not only doesn't reduce the risk of clogged arteries and heart disease (Frantz et al. 1989), it is associated with a disturbing rise in the rates of new cancers (Dayton and Pearce 1969).

Myth: Eating cholesterol increases blood cholesterol levels.

Reality: Dietary cholesterol has essentially no effect on blood cholesterol levels, as the majority of circulating cholesterol does not come from the diet but is manufactured inside the body. So eating a "low-cholesterol" diet in an effort to lower cholesterol is wasted effort (Nelson, Schmidt, and Kelley 1995). But, more importantly, when it comes to the artery-hardening plaques that lead to heart attacks and strokes, we know now that blood cholesterol is not the enemy. The enemies, as it turns out, are small cholesterol-carrying LDL particles that have been oxidized, a process that transforms them from helpful cholesterol scavengers to artery-clogging villains (Holvoet et al. 2001; Holvoet 2004). The best way to generate small, oxidized LDL inside the body, as it turns out, is to eat lots of refined carbohydrates and oxidation-prone omega-6 fatty acids—just the kind of things you'll no longer be doing.

Myth: Whole grains are part of a "balanced diet."

Reality: For almost the entirety of our species' existence on this planet, grains have been unavailable as a food source, as they are toxic to humans when eaten raw. The discovery of methods for rendering them edible was the spark that ignited the agricultural revolution. Grains are nutrient poor and contain substances that block nutrient absorption (phytates), disrupt the intestinal lining (lectins), lead to life-threatening gastrointestinal illness in vulnerable populations, and may be a critical factor in the pathogenesis of a whole host of chronic diseases (gluten).

Myth: This way of eating is "low-carb."

Reality: The standard Western diet is *extraordinarily high* in carbohydrates, thanks to the disproportionate amounts of sugar and wheat flour in it. By comparison, a diet without added sugar and wheat flour will be lower in carbohydrates (since the foods they're replaced with are likely to be higher in fat and protein). The truth is that human beings can thrive on a huge range of macronutrient (protein, fat, carbohydrate) compositions, though in specific circumstances (obesity, diabetes, epilepsy, and chronic migraine) a diet lower in carbohydrates can have therapeutic benefit.

129

Myth: Fat is fat.

Reality: When it comes to the impact of dietary fat on your health, the devil is in the details. Part of the reason things have gotten so confused in the field of nutrition is that we've treated all dietary fat as if it were a single entity, in doing so completely neglecting the fact that the biological effects of fat are entirely dependent on its subtype. Not only has this led to an entire body of scientifically useless nutritional research on the effects of dietary fat, but it has also produced a confusing message to the general public. The reality here is that, even though to many "low fat" is synonymous with "healthy," whether a food item is high in fat or low in fat tells you *absolutely nothing* about whether it is good for you.

KEEPING YOUR MIND RIGHT

Changing lifelong dietary habits is not easy. For some, adopting this diet may require some seemingly radical changes to the way you've been eating. Yet, in my experience, a person's success in transitioning to this way of eating (or in making any significant lifestyle change, for that matter) depends in large part on how you choose to view this change. In particular, it depends on whether you bemoan what's being lost or celebrate what's being gained. Yes, there's no more bread and sugary foods. And there are fewer convenience foods (or "food products") available to you. On the other hand, there are also many wonderful things you may have previously avoided out of a well-intentioned effort to eat "healthy" that you can now eat guilt-free: eggs, bacon, beef, and butter, to name just a few!

To help you maintain your focus on what's important, here's a brief of what you stand to gain by making these changes to your diet:

BENEFITS OF AN ANCESTRAL DIET

- Stable blood sugar levels throughout the day, resulting in stable energy levels, a longer feeling of satiety, elimination of postmeal fatigue and sleepiness, and a more stable mood

- Elimination of bloating and reflux after meals

- Improved blood pressure control

- Misery-free loss of excess body fat

- Significant reduction in your risk of chronic diseases, including diabetes, heart disease, many forms of cancer, arthritis, and general decrepitude

- Guilt-free consumption of large amounts of bacon

AND, last but not least...

- AN END TO MIGRAINES!

If this feels overwhelming to you, commit to doing it for just thirty days and see what happens.

CHAPTER 6

Recipes

Back when I decided to change my way of eating, I was fortunate that my wife, Jenny, was also ready and willing to join me in my efforts. Even better, she was eager to apply her considerable cooking skill and creativity to the task of creating meals for us to enjoy. During the past few years, her efforts have resulted in a diverse and delicious array of recipes. Now you get to enjoy the fruits of that labor as I have!

Without a doubt, there's no better way to ensure a smooth and effective transition to this way of eating than to cook your own food. After all, it's much easier to avoid wheat, hidden sugars, and other potential dietary hazards when you're making your own meals. Yet, for most of you, cooking meals within these guidelines may mean breaking some old habits and starting some new ones. This chapter is here to help get you started.

Many of the recipes use coconut oil as the fat for cooking. Feel free to substitute butter, ghee, olive oil, lard, or other animal fat for the coconut oil if you prefer.

Finally, for carbohydrate counts on each of these recipes (for those of you who are aiming to eat under a certain amount), you'll find them on *The Migraine Miracle* website (www.mymigrainemiracle.com). There, you'll also find even more recipes with which to expand your repertoire.

BREAKFAST

I tend to crave sweet breakfasts over savory, so I've tried to create some recipes that offer the perception of sweetness, though few have any sweeteners. Because spices like cinnamon and cloves and extracts like vanilla, almond, and orange are commonly used in sweet preparations, we associate those flavors with sweetness.

Several recipes in this section call for protein powder. I recommend that you purchase a whey-based protein powder without added sugar. Flavors vary greatly. We suggest that you try multiple brands until you find one that you enjoy. Our favorite happens to be the store brand at our local supermarket.

For additional breakfast ideas, the ancestral health blog Mark's Daily Apple (www.marksdailyapple.com) can be a great resource.

Breakfast Smoothie

This is a quick breakfast that we make most weekday mornings. Not only is it a delicious and satisfying start to the day, but the ketones from the coconut milk will provide you with extra migraine protection.

3 (2-inch) pieces of banana, frozen

7 ounces (about 1 cup) canned coconut milk without guar gum

¼ cup vanilla protein powder

1 tablespoon almond butter

2 tablespoons full-fat Greek yogurt

½ cup ice cubes (optional)

In a blender or smoothie maker, combine all of the ingredients. Blend until smooth and serve.

Makes 1 smoothie

Ricotta Sweet Potato Pancakes

If you have leftover sweet potatoes from dinner, this is a great way to use them up the next morning. Try making bacon before you cook these pancakes and cooking them in the bacon grease. It adds a nice salty/smoky flavor to the cakes.

¾ cup cooked and mashed sweet potato

½ cup almond butter

1 cup whole-milk ricotta cheese

⅛ teaspoon salt

1½ teaspoons ground cinnamon

1 teaspoon baking powder

1½ teaspoons pure vanilla extract

½ cup milk

2 eggs, divided

¼ cup bacon grease

Topping

1 cup heavy whipping cream, cold

1 tablespoon pure vanilla extract

1 cup mixed berries, frozen or fresh

Mix the sweet potato, almond butter, and ricotta cheese in a bowl. Add the salt, cinnamon, and baking powder and mix until just combined.

In another bowl, mix the vanilla, milk, and egg yolks. Then add to the sweet potato mixture.

Beat the reserved egg whites until stiff peaks form. Gently mix two spoonfuls of the whites into the sweet potato mixture. Once incorporated, fold in the remaining egg whites until just combined.

Prepare the whipped cream: Pour the cream and vanilla into the bowl of a stand mixer or a large bowl. Beat the cream until peaks form.

Heat 2 tablespoons of grease in a skillet over medium heat. Spoon the batter into 2- to 3-inch rounds and cook until browned on one side, then flip. Keeping your pancakes small will make them easier to flip. Add more grease to the skillet before spooning in more batter.

To serve, top each pancake with whipped cream and berries.

Makes about 20 small-to-medium pancakes

Southwestern Quiche in a Pepper Bowl

Instead of putting fillings on bread or over pasta, try using veggie "bowls" like hollowed bell peppers, tomatoes, and avocados. These quiches make a great weekend breakfast.

4 red or yellow bell peppers

4 ounces goat cheese

½ cup coarsely chopped onion

½ cup coarsely chopped tomato

2 tablespoons finely chopped jalapeño, seeds intact

2 tablespoons coarsely chopped cilantro

2 cups grated cheddar cheese

6 eggs

1½ cups heavy cream

1 teaspoon salt

½ teaspoon pepper

½ avocado, coarsely chopped

2 tablespoons sour cream

Preheat oven to 325°F.

Core and seed the bell peppers, leaving them otherwise intact. Put 1 ounce goat cheese inside each pepper. Divide the onion, tomato, jalapeño, and cilantro among the four peppers, filling the cavity. Place ¼ cup cheddar on top of the filling inside the pepper.

In a medium bowl, beat the eggs with the cream, salt, and pepper. Pour the egg mixture over the filling inside of the peppers until the peppers are three-fourths full.

Place the peppers on a foil-lined baking pan and bake for 1 hour or until the egg filling is set.

To serve, top each pepper with avocado, sour cream, and the remaining cheddar, divided among the four.

Makes 4 servings

Berries and Cream

Keep a supply of toasted coconut and toasted almonds on hand for quick morning breakfasts. To toast your own nuts, heat them in the oven at 350°F until lightly browned and fragrant (about 10 minutes). For coconut, follow the same method, but reduce the cooking time.

1 cup mixed berries, fresh or frozen

1 tablespoon shredded, unsweetened coconut, toasted

1 tablespoon sliced almonds, toasted

⅛ teaspoon ground cinnamon

⅓ cup half-and-half

Place berries in a small bowl and top with coconut, almonds, and cinnamon. Add cream and stir. Eat immediately or when the berries have thawed.

Makes 1 serving

Chocolate-Orange Nut Bars

I like a sweet grab-and-go breakfast on occasion. Our version of these nut bars was inspired by an energy-bar recipe found on the website Mark's Daily Apple (www.marksdailyapple.com). Of course, they certainly make great snacks, too. To toast your own nuts, heat them in the oven at 350°F until they're lightly browned and fragrant. Follow the same method for coconut, but reduce the cooking time.

½ cup almonds, toasted

½ cup pecans, toasted

½ cup shredded, unsweetened coconut, toasted

½ cup almond butter

¼ cup coconut oil or other recommended fat, heated to a liquid state, plus more to grease the baking dish

2 eggs

1½ teaspoons orange extract

Zest of 1 orange

1 tablespoon honey

1½ teaspoons pure vanilla extract

¼ cup protein powder (optional)

1 ounce 80% dark chocolate (or 70%, if you prefer a sweeter bar), finely chopped

Preheat oven to 325°F. Grease an 8-inch-square baking dish.

In a food processor, finely chop the nuts and coconut. Transfer to a medium bowl and mix in the almond butter and coconut oil.

In a separate small bowl, beat the eggs with the orange extract, zest, honey, and vanilla. Add the egg mixture to the nut mixture and mix well. Stir in the protein powder, if you're using it.

Press the mixture into a prepared dish and top with the chopped chocolate. Bake for 15 minutes and cool before cutting into bars. Store covered for up to 3 to 4 days.

Makes 12 bars

LUNCH

Any of the main dishes can also be made for lunch. I often make extra at dinnertime and eat the leftovers for lunch the next day. It's quite simple to roll up last night's dinner in a lettuce wrap. You can also create a salad with the leftover protein. Just add some cheese and maybe a fruit or nut that you think complements the flavor of the protein. With a drizzle of extra-virgin olive oil and a splash of your favorite vinegar, you'll be set.

Meat and Cheese Roll-Ups

Here's a basic roll-up recipe. Experiment with your favorite ingredients like olives, arugula, or pickles to create your own instant breadless sandwich.

5-ounce round of Boursin cheese

2 tablespoons whipping cream

½ teaspoon salt

6 thick slices Havarti cheese

6 slices deli-style roast beef

3 tablespoons coarsely chopped oil-packed sun-dried tomatoes

3 tablespoons coarsely chopped roasted red peppers

3 tablespoons coarsely chopped avocado

Combine the Boursin cheese, cream, and salt in a small bowl and mix until blended and spreadable.

Lay out the Havarti cheese slices and top each with one slice of roast beef. Spread with the Boursin cheese mixture and top with the remaining ingredients. Roll up the cheese slices and serve. Reserve the remaining Boursin mixture for your next roll-up meal. The mixture should keep for 3 to 4 days.

Makes 6 roll-ups

Smoked-Trout Lettuce Wraps

We typically use smoked trout in this recipe, but you can substitute any smoked fish of your choosing.

Dressing

3 limes, juiced

1 tablespoon raw honey

2 teaspoons gluten-free tamari

1 teaspoon coarse kosher salt

½ teaspoon pepper

Filling

1 cup thinly sliced (into matchsticks) jicama

1 cup cherry tomatoes, halved

½ cup finely chopped fresh basil

½ cup finely chopped fresh mint

¼ cup finely chopped fresh tarragon

1 large shallot, thinly sliced

1 red or orange bell pepper, seeded and chopped

1 hot cherry pepper, chopped, seeds intact

8 ounces smoked trout (or other smoked fish), flaked

1 head Bibb lettuce, leaves separated

To prepare the dressing: In a small bowl, mix the lime juice, honey, and tamari. Add the salt and pepper. Set aside.

To prepare the filling: In a medium bowl, combine the jicama, tomatoes, basil, mint, tarragon, shallot, bell pepper, and cherry pepper. Stir in the dressing.

Lay out lettuce leaves and divide the trout and filling among them. Roll to eat. Serve immediately.

Makes about 8 wraps

Buffalo Chicken with Celery Ribbon and Shaved Carrot Salad

Just like with buffalo wings, you can adjust the heat level of the chicken in this recipe with the amount of sauce you spoon over it when serving.

Chicken

1 stick (½ cup) butter

2 cloves garlic, minced

1 cup hot sauce

2 boneless, skinless chicken breasts, fat trimmed

Salad

2 large carrots, peeled

2 stalks celery, washed and ends trimmed

¼ cup parsley leaves, washed and stemmed

Dressing

3 ounces Maytag blue cheese

2 tablespoons apple cider vinegar

1 teaspoon hot sauce

½ teaspoon salt

¼ cup extra-virgin olive oil

½ cup whipping cream

Preheat oven to 375°F.

In a small saucepan, melt butter with garlic over medium-low heat. Once the butter mixture is melted, remove the pan from the stove and mix in the hot sauce. Cool the mixture slightly.

Place the chicken breasts in an 8-inch-square glass baking dish and top with the sauce mixture. Bake for 30 minutes or until the internal temperature reaches 165°F.

While the chicken is cooking, prepare the salad. Using a vegetable peeler, shave the carrots and celery sticks for the salad. Mix with the parsley leaves.

To prepare the dressing, add the blue cheese, vinegar, hot sauce, and salt to a food processor and pulse to blend. With the processor running, pour in the oil. Once combined, add the cream in the same manner.

To assemble the dish, line plates with the salad and top with dressing. Cut the chicken into ½-inch slices and top the salads with half of a breast on each. Stir the sauce remaining in the glass baking dish, if it has separated, and drizzle it over the chicken. The more sauce you use, the spicier the dish will be.

Makes 4 small salads

Tuna with Pickled Radish

Top pickled radish slices with this Asian-inspired tuna. Having a mandoline slicer to help cut the radish into thin, uniform slices is helpful but not necessary.

Pickled Radish

1 cup rice vinegar

1 tablespoon honey

½ teaspoon salt

1 (1-foot) section of daikon radish, peeled and cut into ⅛-inch-thick horizontal slices

Tuna

1 tuna steak

¼ cup gluten-free tamari

1 clove garlic, minced

1 tablespoon coconut oil or other recommended fat

Dressing

Juice of 2 limes

1 teaspoon Sriracha sauce

1 teaspoon honey

1 teaspoon fresh ginger, peeled and minced

2 teaspoons sesame seeds

Salad

½ cup finely chopped red bell pepper

1 (8-ounce) can water chestnuts, coarsely chopped

¼ cup finely chopped fresh cilantro

In a large, flat bowl, combine vinegar, honey, and salt. Add the radish slices and marinate in the refrigerator for at least an hour. If the slices are not immersed, periodically flip them over in the marinade.

Place the tuna in a bowl or zippered plastic bag. Add the tamari and garlic, and let sit for at least an hour.

While the tuna and radish slices are marinating, prepare the remaining ingredients. Toss the bell pepper, water chestnuts, and cilantro in a small bowl. To make the dressing, combine the limes, Sriracha sauce, and honey in a separate small bowl. Stir in the ginger and sesame seeds.

Heat a skillet with the coconut oil over high heat. Look for waves in the oil to determine when the pan is hot enough. Remove the tuna from the marinade and discard the marinade. Sear the tuna for about 2 minutes per side. The tuna should still be pink in the center when you finish. Allow to cool and slice into ¼-inch-thick pieces.

To assemble the dish, top the radish slices with the salad components and tuna. Drizzle with the dressing.

Makes about 3 servings

Greek Chicken Salad

This is a great make-ahead salad to have for workday lunches. Serve with bell pepper slices or celery sticks.

Chicken

3 boneless, skinless chicken breasts, fat trimmed

½ cup gluten-free tamari

Salt and black pepper

Salad

¼ cup coarsely chopped oil-packed sun-dried tomatoes

1 tablespoon capers, drained

½ cup coarsely chopped Castelvetrano olives, drained

¼ cup coarsely chopped artichoke hearts

3 slices cooked bacon, crumbled (about ½ cup)

2 ounces feta cheese, crumbled

¼ cup full-fat Greek yogurt

½ teaspoon salt

1 tablespoon finely chopped fresh parsley

Preheat oven to 375°F.

Place the chicken breasts in an 8-inch-square glass baking dish and top with the tamari and salt and pepper to taste. Bake for about 30 minutes or until the internal temperature reaches 165°F. Allow to cool.

While the chicken is cooking, combine the tomatoes, capers, olives, artichokes, bacon, and feta in a medium bowl. Add the yogurt, salt, and parsley, and stir until well mixed.

Cut the cooked chicken into 1-inch cubes and add to the salad mixture.

Makes 6 servings

DINNER AND MAIN DISHES

There are a wide variety of main dishes that fit the Miracle diet. Besides the recipes that follow, some basic (slightly modified) standbys to add to your repertoire include stir-fry, grilled link sausage, burgers (try mixing lamb and beef, then pan-frying or grilling, and leave off the bun), and tacos (skip the tortilla and just serve the seasoned meat with lettuce, cheese, sour cream, and salsa).

Grapefruit-Mustard Marinated Lamb

This is a great main dish to serve company. It can also be made on the grill.

Marinade

¾ cup Dijon mustard

2½ cups fresh-squeezed grapefruit juice (about 4 grapefruits)

½ teaspoon ancho chili

½ teaspoon ground allspice

½ teaspoon smoked paprika

¼ teaspoon ground cayenne pepper

2 teaspoons salt

4 cloves garlic, chopped

Lamb

6 lamb loin chops

Salt and pepper

2 tablespoons coconut oil or other recommended fat

8 (2-inch) grapefruit wedges

To make the marinade: Mix the mustard and grapefruit juice in a medium bowl. Stir in the chili powder, allspice, paprika, cayenne pepper, and salt. Add the garlic. Use two-thirds of this mixture to marinate the lamb in a covered dish or zippered plastic bag for at least 30 minutes. Set aside the remaining third of the marinade.

Preheat the broiler.

Remove the lamb from the marinade and season the chops with salt and pepper. Discard the used marinade.

In a grill pan brushed with oil, sear the meat for about 2 minutes per side. Transfer the meat to a roasting pan and add the reserved marinade.

Broil the lamb for 4 to 5 minutes for medium doneness. Flip the meat, top with grapefruit wedges, and broil for another 4 to 5 minutes. Serve topped with grapefruit and pan juices.

Makes 6 servings

Massaman Curry Chicken

Although Thai dishes are often served over rice, if you serve this chicken in a bowl with a spoon, it can be eaten much like a soup. You could also add extra broth and coconut milk to convert it to a true soup. Just be sure to cut the chicken into bite-size pieces.

1 (17-ounce) can coconut milk

⅓ cup chicken broth

⅓ cup cashew butter

1 teaspoon salt

1 teaspoon red pepper flakes, or more for a spicier result

2 tablespoons coconut oil or other recommended fat

3 tablespoons green curry paste

2 tablespoons minced peeled fresh ginger

4 boneless skinless chicken breasts, cubed

1 red bell pepper, seeded and thinly sliced

1 cup finely chopped celery

½ cup sliced green onions, white and light green parts only

½ cup cashews

To make the sauce: In a medium bowl, mix the coconut milk, chicken broth, cashew butter, salt, and red pepper flakes.

Heat the oil in a large sauté pan. Add the curry paste and the ginger. Sauté for 1 to 2 minutes over medium heat until the ginger is fragrant and softening. Add the chicken and cook until the meat is no longer pink. Add the sauce to the pan and continue to cook the chicken over medium-low heat. Add the bell pepper, celery, green onions, and cashews.

Cover and continue to cook for 15 to 20 minutes or until the chicken is cooked throughout. If the sauce becomes too thick, lower the heat and add coconut milk or chicken broth in quarter-cup increments to thin as necessary.

Season to taste with additional salt and red pepper flakes.

Makes 4 servings

Savory Pumpkin Cheesecake

You can have cheesecake for dinner with this savory version. Serve it warm with a side salad. It also reheats well for leftovers.

8 ounces bacon, cooked and crumbled, grease reserved

8 ounces mushrooms, coarsely chopped

1 yellow onion, finely diced

3 cloves garlic, minced

2 tablespoons finely chopped fresh sage, plus 8 whole sage leaves for optional garnish

2 (8-ounce) bricks cream cheese, softened

¼ cup chicken broth

1½ cups pumpkin purée, canned or fresh

½ cup sour cream

4 eggs

1 teaspoon ground allspice

1 teaspoon salt

½ teaspoon pepper

1 cup grated Parmesan cheese, plus more for optional garnish

Ghee, lard, or duck fat, for optional garnish

2 tablespoons roasted and salted pepitas, for optional garnish

Preheat the oven to 300°F.

Grease the bottom and sides of a springform pan with the reserved bacon grease.

In a sauté pan, use 2 tablespoons of the remaining bacon grease to sauté the mushrooms over medium heat for about 3 minutes, or until soft. Remove the mushrooms and spread them in the bottom of the prepared pan to form the crust. Crumble half of the bacon on top of the mushrooms. Set aside.

To prepare the vegetables: Add any remaining bacon grease back to the sauté pan. Add the onion and cook over medium heat for about 5 minutes, or until soft. Add the garlic and chopped sage, and cook for 1 minute more. Remove this mixture and set aside to cool.

To make the filling: In a large bowl, beat the cream cheese, broth, pumpkin, and sour cream with an electric mixer until smooth. Continue beating and add the eggs one at a time until incorporated. Mix in the allspice, salt, and pepper. Fold in the remaining crumbled bacon, Parmesan cheese, and the cooled onion-garlic-sage mixture.

Pour cream cheese–pumpkin filling over the crust and bake for about 70 minutes or until set. Cool for about 20 minutes before serving to allow the cheesecake to firm.

To prepare the garnish (optional): Heat the ghee, lard, or duck fat in a small frying pan over high heat. Drop the whole sage leaves, washed and completely dried, into the oil a few at a time. Fry for a few seconds and carefully remove them with a slotted spoon. Place the leaves on paper towels to drain excess oil.

Garnish the cheesecake with the pepitas, more Parmesan, and the fried sage leaves. Serve warm.

Makes 8 slices

Coconut-Macadamia Salmon with Lime-Butter Sauce

Use the technique of coating different proteins with assorted nuts to create a number of dishes.

Salmon

1 cup macadamia nuts, roasted and salted

½ cup shredded unsweetened coconut

4 salmon fillets

2 tablespoons coconut oil or other recommended fat

Lime-Butter Sauce

8 tablespoons unsalted butter

1 shallot, thinly sliced

¼ cup lime juice

1 teaspoon salt

½ cup cream

Preheat oven to 375°F.

To prepare the salmon: In a food processor, finely chop the nuts and coconut. Brush the salmon with coconut oil and coat with the nut mixture on all sides.

Roast the salmon for 20 minutes. If the nuts brown too quickly, cover loosely with foil.

While the salmon cooks, prepare the sauce: In a saucepan over medium heat, melt the butter and cook the shallot about 2 minutes, or until soft. Add the lime juice and salt, and stir until combined. Add the cream and cook about 5 minutes, until thickened slightly. Serve the salmon topped with sauce.

Makes 4 servings

Grilled Asian Pork Tenderloin

While the pork rests, make a quick vegetable stir-fry with water chestnuts, snow peas, and broccoli to serve with it. For lunch the next day, make a lettuce wrap with the remaining veggies and pork.

1 cup rice wine vinegar

½ cup gluten-free tamari

⅓ cup extra-virgin olive oil

2 tablespoons minced peeled fresh ginger

¼ cup chopped scallions, white and light green parts only

3 cloves garlic, minced

1 pork tenderloin

To prepare marinade: Combine the rice wine vinegar, tamari, olive oil, ginger, scallions, and garlic in a large bowl with a lid. Set aside 1 cup of marinade to use as a sauce. Add the pork to the bowl, cover, and refrigerate. Marinate for 2 to 4 hours.

Preheat grill to medium heat. Remove the tenderloin from the marinade and discard the liquid. Grill the whole tenderloin for about 3 to 4 minutes per side, or until the internal temperature has reached 145°F.

Remove from heat and tent with foil. Allow the pork to rest for about 10 minutes before slicing it to serve. While it rests, heat the reserved marinade over low heat just until warm.

Spoon the sauce over the tenderloin slices and serve.

Makes 4 to 6 servings

Bone Marrow Salad

Many local markets will have marrow bones, but you may have to ask for them to be brought out from the back. You can eat the roasted marrow with a spoon straight from the bone or sprinkle it on a salad as we've suggested here.

Marrow

8 (2- to 3-inch) marrow bones

1 tablespoon finely chopped parsley

2 cloves garlic, minced

1 teaspoon sea salt

Fried capers

½ cup ghee

¼ cup capers, drained and dried

Salad

6 cups arugula

1 shallot, thinly sliced

½ grapefruit, peeled and sectioned

2 teaspoons lemon zest

Extra-virgin olive oil

Juice of two lemons

Sea salt

Preheat oven to 425°F.

Stand the bones on cut ends on a roasting pan. Sprinkle with the parsley, garlic, and salt. Roast for about 20 minutes or until soft enough to spoon marrow out.

While the bones are roasting, fry the capers: Heat the ghee in a small sauté pan over medium-high heat. Test the heat by adding one caper. If it bubbles, the oil is hot enough. Add a spoonful of capers and fry until they begin to color. Remove with a slotted spoon and drain on a paper towel. Repeat with the remaining capers.

To prepare the salad: Divide the arugula among four plates. Top each plate with shallots, grapefruit sections, fried capers, and a sprinkling of lemon zest. Dress each plate with a drizzle of oil and the juice of half a lemon. Spoon bits of bone marrow onto each salad and top with a sprinkle of sea salt. Serve immediately.

Makes 4 servings

Sage Pork Chops with Brown Butter Sauce

This simple recipe highlights the flavor of great chops.

Chops

4 bone-in pork chops

4 tablespoons fresh sage, finely chopped

Salt and pepper

3 tablespoons ghee

Sauce

6 tablespoons unsalted butter

1 teaspoon salt

3 tablespoons cream

Pat the chops dry and sprinkle with sage, salt, and pepper.

Heat the ghee in a sauté pan over medium-high heat until hot. Add the pork chops and brown on each side for about 3 minutes. If you try to flip the meat and it sticks, it isn't ready. Transfer the chops to a plate and tent with foil while you prepare the sauce.

In a small saucepan, melt the butter over medium-low heat and cook until it begins to color. Watch it carefully, as it will burn quickly. Once the butter has started to brown, add the salt and cream. Stir and cook for another 4 to 5 minutes until slightly thickened.

Spoon the sauce over the chops and serve.

Makes 4 servings

Cilantro-Lime Shrimp

Make this a meal with grilled veggies. Choose your favorite vegetables—onions, bell peppers, and mushrooms are excellent choices—and grill them on skewers. Drizzle with olive oil and lime to serve.

½ cup lime juice

Zest of 2 limes

1 cup extra-virgin olive oil

4 cloves garlic, minced

¼ cup cilantro, finely chopped

1 pound jumbo shrimp (21–24 whole shrimp), peeled and deveined

Wooden skewers, soaked in water for at least an hour

Salt and pepper

Combine lime juice, lime zest, olive oil, garlic, and cilantro in a small bowl. Place the marinade and shrimp into a large zippered plastic bag and refrigerate. Marinate for 2 hours.

Preheat grill.

Remove the shrimp from the marinade, and discard the remaining liquid. Thread shrimp onto skewers and sprinkle with salt and pepper.

Grill over medium heat for 1 to 2 minutes per side. Serve immediately.

Makes 4 to 5 servings

Pecan Chicken with Mustard Sauce

Make this recipe even more kid-friendly by substituting chicken tenders for the breasts. Prepare a quick honey-mustard dip for the kiddos using two parts Greek yogurt to one part honey and one part mustard.

Chicken

3 tablespoons coconut oil or other recommended fat

2 cups pecans, finely chopped

1 teaspoon salt

1 teaspoon pepper

6 boneless, skinless chicken breasts, fat trimmed

1 egg, lightly beaten

Mustard Sauce

½ cup heavy cream

1 cup Dijon mustard

½ teaspoon salt

2 tablespoons apple cider vinegar

2 tablespoons unsalted butter

Preheat the oven to 375°F.

To prepare the chicken: Heat the oil in a sauté pan over medium-high heat. While it's heating, combine the pecans, salt, and pepper in a shallow bowl or plate. Dip the chicken in the egg and then coat with the pecan mixture on all sides.

Add the chicken to the sauté pan and brown about 2 to 3 minutes per side. Transfer to a glass baking dish and bake for about 25 minutes or until cooked through. If the pecans begin to brown too rapidly, cover with foil. *Note: If you are using pounded breasts or cutlets, the cooking time will be shortened.*

To prepare the sauce: Mix the cream, mustard, and salt in a small saucepan over medium-low heat. Simmer until slightly thickened, about 5 to 7 minutes. Add the vinegar and butter, and stir until melted. Remove from heat. Pour onto the cooked chicken and serve immediately.

Makes 6 servings

Sausage and Veggies Bake

We usually make this dish about once a week to use any vegetables remaining from our weekly vegetable box from a local farm. The two key components are the chorizo sausage and sweet potatoes, but any other vegetables can be substituted or added.

  1 pound bulk chorizo sausage

  2 sweet potatoes, peeled and cut into ½-inch cubes

  2 red or yellow bell peppers, seeded and cut into 1-inch pieces

  1 red onion, cut into 1-inch pieces

  1 bunch asparagus, cut into 1-inch pieces

  2 cups snow peas

  3 teaspoons salt

  2 cloves garlic, minced

Preheat oven to 375°F.

Brown the sausage in a sauté pan over medium heat and set aside.

Add sweet potatoes, peppers, onion, asparagus, and snow peas to a roasting pan and pour the sausage (including the pan grease) over the top. Mix together and add salt.

Cook for 25 minutes, stirring every 10 to 15 minutes. After 30 minutes, stir in the garlic and cook for another 10 minutes or until the vegetables are tender.

  Serves 4 to 6

Crab and Tomato Ragout

We often make this recipe the same week that we make the Crab Cakes to use any remaining crab. It can be eaten alone or served inside bell pepper or avocado vegetable bowls.

3 tablespoons coconut oil or other recommended fat

2 leeks, white and light green parts halved and sliced

2 cloves garlic, minced

1 jalapeño pepper, chopped, seeds intact

2 cups seeded and chopped tomatoes

3 tablespoons apple cider vinegar

3 teaspoons salt

½ pound jumbo lump crab, picked through for shells

Heat the oil in a sauté pan over medium heat. Add leeks and cook for about 3 minutes, until they start to soften. Add the garlic and jalapeño, and cook for another minute. Add the tomatoes, vinegar, and salt. Simmer for about 5 minutes and add the crab. Cook for another 2 minutes. Serve warm.

Makes 3 to 4 servings

Eggplant and Sausage Lasagna

This is a noodle-less lasagna that uses the eggplant to form the layers. This recipe precooks the eggplant, enhancing its flavor and speeding the final baking time. This is a good meal to prepare ahead and stick in the oven to warm before serving.

   1 large eggplant, peeled and sliced into ¼-inch-thick rounds

   6 tablespoons olive oil

   3 teaspoons salt

   5 tablespoons balsamic vinegar

   ½ yellow onion, coarsely chopped

   2 cloves garlic, minced

   1 (28-ounce) can San Marzano tomatoes (should already be crushed and peeled)

   ½ cup chicken stock

   ½ pound Italian sausage, cooked crumbled if in bulk or cooked and sliced if in links

   8 ounces fresh mozzarella cheese, cut into ½-inch-thick slices

   2 cups grated mozzarella cheese

   2 tablespoons finely chopped fresh basil

Preheat oven to 375°F.

Toss the eggplant slices with 3 tablespoons of the oil, 1 teaspoon of the salt, and 3 tablespoons of the vinegar. Set aside.

Coat a large saucepan with 1 tablespoon of the remaining olive oil and heat over medium-high heat. Add the onion and cook for about 5 minutes. Add the garlic and continue to cook for another 5 minutes. Add the remaining 2 tablespoons vinegar, the tomatoes, and the stock. Simmer for 10 to 15 minutes, until thickened and half of the liquid has evaporated. Set aside.

Cook the eggplant in a large sauté pan over medium heat. Add 1 table-spoon oil at a time as needed to coat the pan. Cook the eggplant slices on each side until soft, about 5 minutes per side. The eggplant may need to be cooked in batches.

Brush a 3-quart rectangular baking dish with 1 tablespoon olive oil. Layer with the eggplant, tomato sauce, cheeses, sausage, and basil. Reserve enough shredded mozzarella to cover the top layer.

Bake for about 20 minutes, or until heated through and top layer of cheese has browned. Serve warm.

Makes about 8 servings

Crab Cakes

When forming these, try to leave the crab lumpy so you don't end up with a stringy crab cake.

   2 cups pecans

   2/3 cup grated Parmesan

   1 teaspoon finely chopped parsley

   ½ cup Dijon mustard

   1 egg

   1 teaspoon hot sauce

   ½ teaspoon apple cider vinegar

   1 teaspoon salt

   12 ounces jumbo lump crab, picked through for shells

   2 tablespoons coconut oil or other recommended fat

In a food processor, pulse 1 cup of the pecans with the Parmesan and parsley until finely ground and blended. (If you don't have a food processor, chop the ingredients by hand and combine.) Set aside.

Chop the remaining 1 cup pecans in the food processor until finely ground and set aside on a plate.

In a separate medium bowl, combine the mustard, egg, hot sauce, vinegar, and salt. Incorporate the Parmesan-pecan mixture. Fold in the crab gently, taking care not to break up the crab.

Scoop into 2- to 3-inch mounds and coat with ground pecans.

Heat 1 tablespoon of the oil in a medium sauté pan over medium heat. Cook the crab cakes for 3 to 4 minutes per side or until browned. Add more oil as needed to coat the pan. Serve warm.

Serving suggestion: If you'd prefer to serve the crab cakes with a sauce, the Mustard Sauce that accompanies the Pecan Chicken would be an appropriate pairing.

   Makes 8 to 10 cakes

SIDE DISHES AND SNACKS

For accompanying side dishes, we recommend roasted vegetables. Roasting is one of the easiest and tastiest ways to prepare nature's bounty. For most vegetables, we toss with some oil, salt, and pepper and roast at 400°F until al dente. Here are a few vegetables to roast, along with a few other items to add to the mix:

- Brussels sprouts, halved and outer leaves separated; add bacon, cheese, or toasted nuts to roasted sprouts

- Green beans with garlic; after roasting add crumbled bacon and grated Parmesan cheese

- Asparagus

- New potatoes, cubed with rosemary

- Sweet potatoes, cubed

- Kale

Roasted Beet Salad

This salad is quite simple to prepare, but roasting the beets takes a bit of time. Roast them in advance and refrigerate them until the rest of the salad is ready to assemble. To toast your own pecans, heat them in the oven at 350°F until they're lightly browned and fragrant This will take about 10 minutes.

> 2 cups peeled and chopped (into 1-inch cubes) beets
>
> 2 tablespoons olive oil
>
> 1 teaspoon salt
>
> ½ cup pecans, toasted
>
> 2 ounces goat cheese, crumbled

Preheat oven to 400°F.

Lay out two pieces of overlapping foil and top with the chopped beets. Drizzle the beets with olive oil and sprinkle with salt. Wrap the foil pieces around the beets to create a packet and place on a baking sheet. Cook about 1 hour, or until tender.

Let cool, then toss with toasted pecans and goat cheese crumbles.

Makes 4 side servings

Roasted Cherry Tomatoes

We love this recipe so much that we grow cherry tomatoes on our deck each summer just so that we have an ample supply to make it often.

    2 cups cherry (or other miniature) tomatoes

    2 tablespoons olive oil

    1 teaspoon salt

    2 cloves garlic, minced

    ½ cup grated Parmesan cheese

    1 tablespoon finely chopped fresh basil

Preheat oven to 375°F.

In a medium bowl, toss the cherry tomatoes with the olive oil and salt. Place the tomatoes on a roasting pan and roast for about 15 minutes. Sprinkle the garlic onto the pan and roast for another 10 minutes, or until tomatoes pop and garlic begins to brown.

Remove the tomatoes from the oven and transfer them, with the pan drippings, to the same bowl. Toss with Parmesan and basil and serve warm.

    Makes 4 side servings

Turnip "Mac & Cheese"

Here's a grown-up version of a macaroni and cheese dish. This cheesy bacon-studded version is made with turnips in place of pasta. It is substantial enough that it can be served as a side or main dish.

> 6 slices of bacon, cooked and chopped or crumbled, grease reserved
>
> 3 cups heavy cream
>
> 3 tablespoons unsalted butter
>
> 1 tablespoon dry mustard
>
> 1½ teaspoons salt
>
> 1 egg
>
> 6 cups peeled and grated turnips
>
> 1½ cups grated Parmesan cheese
>
> 2 cups grated Gruyère cheese

Preheat oven to 375°F. Grease a 3-quart rectangular baking dish with the reserved bacon drippings.

Combine the cream, butter, mustard, and salt in a pot and bring to a simmer (do not boil). Meanwhile, in a large bowl, lightly beat the egg. When the cream has simmered, temper the eggs by adding a spoonful of the warm cream to the egg, stirring immediately. Continue stirring as you add cream by the spoonful until the egg mixture is warm to the touch. Once warm, incorporate the remaining cream mixture into the egg mixture. Set aside.

Begin layering ingredients. Spread about 2 cups of the turnips over the bottom of the baking dish. Add about one-third of the bacon on top, then ladle one-third of the egg and cream mixture over that, then top with about one-third of each of the two cheeses. Continue layering with the remaining ingredients to build two additional layers.

Bake for 45 to 55 minutes, or until turnips are soft. If the top browns too quickly, cover with foil. Serve warm.

Makes 8 to 10 servings

Squash Cakes

Here's a hearty side dish that will make an appropriate accompaniment to most entrées. The key to making these is in coating the outside of the cakes well so that the cheese will crisp up as it fries, sealing in the soft squash mixture.

> 2 tablespoons coconut oil or other recommended fat
>
> ½ yellow onion, finely chopped
>
> 2 cloves garlic, minced
>
> ½ cayenne pepper, finely chopped with seeds and ribs included
>
> 2 squash (such as Delicata), roasted, scooped, and mashed (about 3 cups)
>
> 1 cup shredded Parmigiano-Reggiano cheese
>
> 1 teaspoon salt
>
> 1 tablespoon fresh parsley, finely chopped

Add 1 tablespoon of the oil to a large sauté pan and sauté the onion over medium heat for about 5 minutes. Add the garlic and pepper, and sauté about 5 more minutes until soft and fragrant. Remove from heat and cool in a large bowl.

Add the squash, ½ cup of the cheese, salt, and parsley to the onion mixture. Form into loose 2- to 3-inch patties, and coat the outsides with the remaining cheese.

Heat the remaining tablespoon of oil in the same saucepan over medium heat. Cook the squash cakes for about 4 to 5 minutes per side or until the cheese has browned on both sides.

Makes about 6 to 8 cakes

Arugula-Pesto Deviled Eggs

Deviled eggs can be a blank canvas for nearly any flavor combination. Play around and turn your favorite recipes into deviled egg recipes. The possibilities are endless. We've included one of our standards to get you started. To toast the pine nuts it calls for, heat them in the oven at 350°F until they're lightly browned and fragrant.

1 dozen eggs, hard-boiled

4 cups arugula

¼ cup extra-virgin olive oil

1 cup grated Parmesan cheese

½ cup pine nuts, toasted

2 tablespoons lemon juice

2 cloves garlic

½ cup crème fraîche

½ teaspoon salt

12 grapefruit sections, peeled and halved

Cut the eggs in half lengthwise and remove the yolks. Add the yolks to a medium bowl and set aside.

To prepare the pesto: Combine the arugula, olive oil, ½ cup of the Parmesan, pine nuts, lemon juice, and garlic in a food processor and pulse until the ingredients are puréed, forming a paste. Set aside.

To prepare the filling: Add the crème fraîche to the egg yolks and mix until smooth. Stir in ¾ cup of the pesto and salt. Reserve the rest of the pesto in the refrigerator for another use. Add the filling to either a pastry bag fitted with a large round tip or a zippered plastic bag with one corner snipped off. Pipe into the hollow egg whites.

To garnish: Top the eggs with grapefruit sections and a sprinkling of the remaining Parmesan.

Makes 24 deviled eggs

Sausage-Stuffed Mushrooms

These filled mushrooms are really versatile. They work well as an appetizer, but they're hearty enough as a main dish served with a side salad. Simply adjust the cooking time depending on the size of mushroom you use.

12 whole portobellini mushrooms

1 round garlic & herbs Boursin cheese or other herbed cream cheese

¼ cup whipping cream

1 teaspoon salt

¼ cup oil-packed sun-dried tomatoes, drained and coarsely chopped

¼ cup coarsely chopped roasted red peppers

1 pound bulk Italian sausage, cooked, drained, and cooled

¾ cup spinach leaves, stemmed and torn into roughly 1-inch pieces (no need to be precise)

Preheat the oven to 400°F.

To prepare the mushrooms: Brush the mushrooms clean, core, and remove the stems.

To prepare the filling: In a medium bowl mix the Boursin cheese and whipping cream until softened. Mix in the salt. Incorporate the tomatoes, peppers, and sausage into the cheese mixture. Fold in the spinach.

Fill the mushroom cavities with the stuffing mixture and bake on a foil-lined sheet pan for about 20 minutes, or until the mushrooms are wilted and the filling is slightly browned and warm to the touch.

Makes 12 mushrooms

Kale Chips

If you ever wondered what to do with kale, here you go. These chips are quite addictive and make a great stand-in when you have the munchies.

1 bunch kale, washed and well-dried

¼ cup extra virgin olive oil

2 teaspoons kosher salt

Preheat the oven to 350°F and line a sheet pan with aluminum foil.

To prepare the kale: remove the thick stems from the middle and tear into 2- to 3-inch pieces. In a medium bowl, toss with the olive oil and salt, coating each leaf. Spread evenly on the baking sheet.

Bake until all of the leaves are crispy, about 15 minutes. Pull the pan out to toss the leaves once over the course of baking, to ensure even cooking. Be sure to taste a chip or two to test for crispness before removing the pan from the oven.

Makes about 4 servings

Macadamia Mascarpone Cheese Log

This slightly sweet cheese log pairs well with celery and other raw vegetables. Toast hte shredded coconut by heating it in the oven at 350°F until it's lightly browned and fragrant. This won't take long—less than 10 minutes.

8 ounces mascarpone cheese, at room temperature

3 teaspoons lemon juice (about 1 lemon)

Zest of 1 lemon

2 teaspoons honey

¾ cup macadamia nuts

¾ cup shredded unsweetened coconut, toasted

In a medium bowl, mix together the cheese, lemon juice, zest, and honey. On a serving dish, form the cheese into a log or mound.

In a food processor, finely chop the macadamia nuts and coconut together. Gently press on to the top and sides of the cheese log to coat.

Serves 8

DESSERT

In all likelihood, after transitioning to this way of eating and freeing your taste buds from the gustatory assault of modern convenience foods, you will find that your affinity for sugary foods pretty much disappears. You'll appreciate a natural sweetness in certain foods that you never knew existed, and you'll also find that most traditional desserts you once thought delicious now taste cloyingly sweet (and you'll wonder how on earth you ever thought soda tasted good!). This shift in your palate will, on the whole, obviate the need for a "dessert course" in your meal. Yet there still may be the occasional time when you need to make something within this dietary framework that will fulfill the dessert role, and that's what this section is for.

Toasted Coconut Cocoa Rounds

While they may sound sweet, these little bites only give the illusion of sweetness with the cocoa. NTo toast your own nuts, heat them in the oven at 350°F until lightly browned and fragrant (about 10 minutes). For coconut, follow the same method, but reduce the cooking time.

½ cup almond butter

1 teaspoon coconut oil or other recommended fat

1 tablespoon unsweetened cocoa powder

1½ cups shredded unsweetened coconut, toasted

Combine the almond butter and oil in a small bowl. Mix in the cocoa.

Drop mixture by teaspoons into a bowl of the coconut and gently roll into balls, coating in coconut. Refrigerate about an hour or until firm.

Makes about 16 rounds

Mixed-Berry Custards

These custards can be eaten warm straight from the oven or refrigerated and served cold. Make them in advance for a quick breakfast, snack, or dessert.

Coconut oil or other recommended fat to grease ramekins

2 eggs

1 cup heavy cream

1 teaspoon cinnamon

1 teaspoon vanilla extract

2 cups mixed berries, fresh or thawed, drained

Preheat oven to 325°F. Grease four custard cups or ramekins with some coconut oil and set aside.

Lightly beat the eggs in a small bowl and set aside.

Stir the cream, cinnamon, and vanilla together in a small saucepan, and bring to a simmer over low heat. Do not allow to boil. Once warmed, add a spoonful of this warm cream mixture to the eggs and mix thoroughly. Continue stirring warm spoonfuls of cream into the eggs until the egg mixture is warm to the touch. Incorporate the remainder of the cream mixture into the eggs.

Fill the greased custard cups or ramekins with the custard. Spoon berries into each. Note that the custard itself is not sweetened. The berries will provide all of the sweetness, so be sure not to skimp on the berries.

Bake for about 35 minutes or until set. Serve warm or cold.

Makes 4 custards

Pecan Sandies

These cookies remind me of pecan sandies in texture and of graham crackers in flavor. While they are tasty right off the pan, we actually prefer them once they have cooled.

1 cup pecan meal (made by grinding pecans in a food processor or nut mill)

¼ cup tapioca flour

¼ teaspoon baking powder

1 tablespoon honey

½ stick (¼ cup) butter, softened

1 teaspoon pure vanilla extract

18 whole pecans

Preheat oven to 350°F and line a baking sheet with parchment paper.

In a medium bowl, combine the pecan meal, tapioca flour, and baking powder. In a separate small bowl, combine the honey, butter, and vanilla. Add the butter mixture to the pecan mixture and stir until incorporated.

Using a 1-inch cookie scoop, spoon the cookies onto the baking sheet, spacing them about 2 inches apart. Press a whole pecan into the center of each cookie, flattening them slightly as you do so.

Bake for about 12 minutes or until cookies begin to brown around the edges.

Makes 1½ dozen

Frozen Banana Pops

This makes a nice summer treat. Enlist the kids to help make them. To toast the coconut, heat it in the oven at 350°F until it's lightly browned and fragrant.

    3 small bananas

    6 popsicle sticks

    8 ounces 80% dark chocolate (or 70%, if you prefer a sweeter flavor), coarsely chopped

    1 tablespoon coconut oil or other recommended fat

    ¼ cup nuts (optional)

    ¼ cup shredded unsweetened coconut, toasted (optional)

Break bananas into 3-inch sections. Insert popsicle sticks halfway into the banana and freeze for at least 3 hours.

Simmer water in the bottom of a double boiler over low heat. In the top bowl, gently melt the chocolate with the coconut oil, stirring often. Once melted, tilt the bowl to the side and dip the banana sections in the chocolate. Immediately sprinkle with desired toppings like nuts or coconut, before the chocolate hardens. Return the bananas to the freezer briefly if they do not harden completely.

    Makes 6 servings

CHAPTER 7

21-Day Meal Plan

"Just tell me exactly what to eat" is a refrain I've heard from folks on more than one occasion after they've learned of the benefits of this way of eating. They understand the rationale and are ready to make the change, but they're still intimidated by those first few steps. This chapter is for them: a no-frills meal plan that walks you through the first three weeks of the transition to an ancestral diet. By following the plan laid out here, you'll be making your first steps toward a migraine-free future, and you'll be building habits that will help ensure success beyond the first three weeks.

I realize that many of you may have time constraints in the morning (as I do), and so breakfast typically contains at least one quick-to-prepare option. You'll find that, in many instances (weekdays in particular), lunch consists of leftovers from the night before. Depending on how much you have left over, you may be able to use these for several lunches in a row, and you may even wish to reheat leftovers for dinner.

Feel free to follow this meal plan exactly as written or modify it to fit your own needs.

WEEK 1

Day 1

Breakfast: Breakfast Smoothie or sausage/bacon and eggs

Lunch: Meat and Cheese Roll-Ups

Dinner: Pecan Chicken with Mustard Sauce

Day 2

Breakfast: Breakfast Smoothie or sausage/bacon and eggs

Lunch: Pecan Chicken with Mustard Sauce (leftovers), either alone or as part of a salad or lettuce wrap

Dinner: Grilled Asian Pork Tenderloin with roasted asparagus

Day 3

Breakfast: Breakfast Smoothie or sausage/bacon and eggs

Lunch: Grilled Asian Pork Tenderloin (leftovers), either alone or as part of a salad or lettuce wrap

Dinner: Massaman Curry Chicken

Day 4

Breakfast: Breakfast Smoothie or sausage/bacon and eggs

Lunch: Massaman Curry Chicken (leftovers), either as is or thinned with coconut milk to make a soup

Dinner: Burger patty (with or without cheese) with Roasted Cherry Tomatoes

Day 5

Breakfast: Breakfast Smoothie or sausage/bacon and eggs

Lunch: Burger patty with Roasted Cherry Tomatoes (leftovers)

Dinner: Sage Pork Chops with Brown Butter Sauce and roasted Brussels sprouts

Day 6 (weekend)

Breakfast: Breakfast Smoothie or Southwestern Quiche in a Pepper Bowl

Lunch: Buffalo Chicken with Celery Ribbon and Shaved Carrot Salad

Dinner: Grapefruit-Mustard Marinated Lamb with roasted sweet potatoes

Day 7 (weekend)

Breakfast: Breakfast Smoothie or scrambled eggs

Lunch: Grapefruit-Mustard Marinated Lamb (leftovers), either alone or as part of a salad or lettuce wrap

Dinner: Cilantro-Lime Shrimp with skewers of grilled bell peppers and onions

WEEK 2

Before this week begins, make a batch of the Chocolate-Orange Nut Bars to have for the upcoming week. These will provide an additional breakfast option and a convenient snack, if needed.

Day 8

Breakfast: Breakfast Smoothie or Chocolate-Orange Nut Bar

Lunch: Cilantro-Lime Shrimp (leftovers), either alone or as part of a salad or lettuce wrap

Dinner: Pecan Chicken with Mustard Sauce and roasted green beans

Day 9

Breakfast: Breakfast Smoothie or Chocolate-Orange Nut Bar

Lunch: Pecan Chicken with Mustard Sauce (leftovers), either alone or as part of a salad or lettuce wrap

Dinner: Sausage-Stuffed Mushrooms with a side salad

Day 10

Breakfast: Breakfast Smoothie or Chocolate-Orange Nut Bar

Lunch: Sausage-Stuffed Mushrooms (leftovers)

Dinner: Crab Cakes with roasted asparagus

Day 11

Breakfast: Breakfast Smoothie or Chocolate-Orange Nut Bar

Lunch: Crab Cake (leftovers) made into a salad

Dinner: Beef, chicken, or shrimp stir-fry

Day 12

Breakfast: Breakfast Smoothie or Chocolate-Orange Nut Bar

Lunch: Beef, chicken, or shrimp stir-fry (leftovers)

Dinner: Crab and Tomato Ragout with roasted crispy kale

Day 13 (weekend)

Breakfast: Berries and Cream

Lunch: Greek Chicken Salad

Dinner: Sausage and Veggies Bake

Day 14 (weekend)

Breakfast: Ricotta Sweet Potato Pancakes

Lunch: Sausage and Veggies Bake (leftovers)

Dinner: Pecan Chicken with Mustard Sauce

WEEK 3

Day 15

Breakfast: Breakfast Smoothie or Berries and Cream

Lunch: Arugula-Pesto Deviled Eggs

Dinner: Eggplant and Sausage Lasagna

Day 16

Breakfast: Breakfast Smoothie or Berries and Cream

Lunch: Eggplant and Sausage Lasagna (leftovers)

Dinner: Savory Pumpkin Cheescake with side salad

Day 17

Breakfast: Breakfast Smoothie or Berries and Cream

Lunch: Savory Pumpkin Cheesecake (leftovers)

Dinner: Massaman Curry Chicken

Day 18

Breakfast: Breakfast Smoothie or Berries and Cream

Lunch: Massaman Curry Chicken (leftovers), either as is or thinned with coconut milk to make a soup

Dinner: Taco meat with lettuce, cheese, sour cream, avocado, and salsa

Day 19

Breakfast: Breakfast Smoothie or Berries and Cream

Lunch: Taco meat with lettuce, cheese, sour cream, avocado, and salsa (leftovers)

Dinner: Coconut-Macadamia Salmon with Lime-Butter Sauce and green beans

Day 20 (weekend)

Breakfast: Ricotta Sweet Potato Pancakes or Berries and Cream

Lunch: Tuna with Pickled Radish

Dinner: Sage Pork Chops with Brown Butter Sauce and Squash Cakes

Day 21 (weekend)

Breakfast: Ricotta Sweet Potato Pancakes or Berries and Cream

Lunch: Sage Pork Chops with Brown Butter Sauce (leftovers), either alone or as part of a salad or lettuce wrap

Dinner: Grilled sausage with Turnip "Mac & Cheese"

CHAPTER 8

Frequently Asked Questions

As you proceed along your journey to adopt an ancestral diet, questions are bound to arise. In my efforts to help family, friends, and patients through this process, I've found that certain questions commonly crop up. In this chapter, I'll review the ones I encounter most often. For each question, I've provided both a short and to-the-point answer and a longer, more nuanced explanation.

If you don't find an answer to what you're looking for in this section, you can also consult the Migraine Miracle website at www.mymigraine miracle.com. You might find the answer to your question in the content that's already there, or you can post your question in the user forum.

I eat out a good bit, but it seems like the only way to eat like this is to prepare my own meals. Is that the case?

Short Answer: Preparing your own meals is the single best way to take control of your health.

Long Answer: You're right; you will find it much easier to eat this way if you are preparing your own meals. For those used to doing so, shifting to an ancestral diet will simply mean shifting the contents of your grocery list and pantry. For those of you not used to cooking for yourselves, adopting this way of eating may seem intimidating or unrealistic. Though it is possible to eat out and for the most part still adhere to the guidelines (see next question), I encourage you to do everything in your power to work toward making as much food for yourself as possible.

To be sure, one of the fundamental reasons that we're suffering from so many diet-related diseases as a society is because we're often not involved in the process of producing the food we eat. For if we don't fully appreciate or understand what it is we put inside our bodies day in and day out, how can we appreciate its impact on our health or the way we feel? And how can we expect to make good decisions about the food we eat if we don't even really know what's in it? In many ways, losing touch with the process of preparing our own food has also caused us to lose touch with the very fact that, more than anything else, what we eat is what determines our health and well-being. Without a doubt, if today everyone started simply preparing their own meals using whole foods, rates of chronic disease would soon plummet, and our health care crisis would become a distant memory.

If you're worried because you have little experience in the kitchen, fear not. Eating this way does not demand any refined cooking techniques, nor does it require hours of work in the kitchen. In fact, one of the benefits of eating this way is that your meals can be prepared simply and quickly, yet the results will be delicious and satisfying. Real food just tastes better.

If you're worried about the demands of a busy schedule, focus on things you can make in large quantities ahead of time that will provide several days' worth of leftovers, and things you can make when you have the time and then freeze for later. If you make this a priority, you'll find ways to make it happen. And you won't be sorry.

How do I maintain this way of eating when I eat out?

Short Answer: You can make it work for the most part, with perhaps some small compromises.

Long Answer: Without a doubt, it's much easier to maintain control of your diet when you're cooking for yourself, and there's no better way to appreciate what's going into your body than to prepare your own food. That said, there will of course be times when you'll either want or need to eat out, and remaining faithful to this way of eating may seem more difficult. But fear not. As I wrote in chapter 5, the most important objective is to avoid wheat flour and added sugar. Though this may require passing on the bread basket or skipping the dessert course, you should still find plenty of suitable options.

Furthermore, the growing recognition of the prevalence of gluten-intolerant and -sensitive diners has led to an ever-expanding number of gluten-free options gracing restaurant menus. Many restaurants now maintain a separate gluten-free menu, so don't be afraid to ask if one is available. Furthermore, as awareness about the health dangers of wheat flour and gluten in particular continues to grow, the marketplace will continue to respond. Slowly but surely we're moving toward a bread-free future, which will only make it easier and easier to find healthy options at your favorite restaurant.

I'm married to a food critic, so I eat out quite a bit. Yet I've found it quite easy to remain compliant with this way of eating while serving as her primary dining companion.

The one area you have little control over is the type of cooking oil used in the food's preparation. In this case, there's little we can do but accept that we may be exposed to more omega-6 in our meal than we'd like. In my opinion, this is an acceptable compromise. Remember, the primary reason for avoiding vegetable and seed oils is to limit consumption of proinflammatory n-6 polyunsaturated fats (PUFAs), whose excess in relation to omega-3 fatty acids leads to chronic systemic inflammation. Though this isn't something you'd want to make a habit of, an occasional day of excess PUFA isn't the worst thing. Furthermore, on days when your meal may contain some unwanted cooking oils, you can help mitigate the consequences by supplementing with a dose of omega-3 (i.e., fish oil) to keep the 6:3 ratio closer to the ideal.

How long will it be before I start seeing results?

Short Answer: Two days to two weeks, depending largely on your pre-transition diet.

Long Answer: The time it takes to experience the full protection against migraines from an ancestral diet will vary from person to person. In large part, this will depend on how you used to eat, as that will determine how significant the metabolic transition will be for your body. For some, the benefits will begin in a matter of days and continue from then on. A minority of folks, particularly those whose pre-transition diet has been high in refined carbohydrates (white flour, sugar, processed foods), may experience some withdrawal-like symptoms during the first week or two. Most who have this experience report feelings of malaise and mental cloudiness—signs that your body is still shifting to its fat-burning machinery and ramping up glucose synthesis in the liver to meet the energy demands of the body and brain. For some, these symptoms may also include headaches, and a small minority may even experience an increase in headache frequency for the first two weeks of the transition.

Once the metabolic transition is complete, these symptoms will disappear, and the protection against migraine will begin.

I just started eating like this and am finding that I'm still getting hungry between meals. What should I do?

Short Answer: Increase the amount of quality fat or protein in your meals.

Long Answer: As discussed in chapter 5, one of the natural consequences of an ancestral diet is that your body will shift its primary energy source from *glucocentric* (sugar) to *adipocentric* (fat). When this happens, you will notice a dramatic stabilization in your energy and hunger levels. However, this shift in metabolism doesn't happen immediately, on average taking roughly two weeks or so of adherence to an ancestral diet to occur completely. One of the hallmarks of a sugar-centric metabolism is the roller coaster of energy levels and, relatedly, hunger and satiety that characterizes day-to-day experience. In this state, the body is dependent on frequent hits of sugar/carbohydrates to supply its energy needs. As the hours pass from the last meal, the blood sugar drops and the brain senses a need for the next hit of sugar. Though there is typically plenty of energy stored away in the adipose tissue, it isn't readily accessible.

Once the shift from glucocentric to adipocentric metabolism is complete, however, most folks will find it quite easy to go extended periods of time without food. Your body is no longer dependent on the next burst of dietary sugar. In this case, as the hours pass from the last meal, the adipose tissue begins releasing stored fat into the bloodstream, maintaining a steady supply of energy for the body's operation. If you need to snack between meals during this transitional phase, that is perfectly fine, just aim for either high-fat or high-protein options. Good choices for snacks include:

- Protein bars (see recipe for Chocolate-Orange Nut Bars in chapter 6)

- Nuts (macadamias are best; almonds, walnuts, and pecans are also good choices)

- High-fat dairy: whole milk, coffee with cream, Greek yogurt *without* the fat removed (add berries or dried fruit if desired), soft cheeses

- Cured meats

- Dark chocolate (70% cocoa or more)

Just remember not to reach for a piece of fruit or the blood sugar spike may well provoke a migraine!

If you've passed beyond the two-week mark and are still noticing hunger between meals, you may just not be eating enough with each meal. For folks eating a typical Western diet, eliminating flour and sugar means eliminating the primary source of calories in their diet. As a result, some other foods will take the place of those lost calories. Some of you may end up increasing your vegetable consumption a good bit, which overall is a wonderful thing. But most vegetables are not particularly energy dense—a nice helping of spinach has only 15 calories, while a single slice of white bread has 65. So if you find yourself getting hungry between meals, try adding in some energy-dense foods with your meals like meats, eggs, fish, high-fat dairy, nuts, cheese, olive oil, coconut (including coconut oil or milk), and sweet potatoes/yams.

What happens if I cheat?

Short Answer: Enjoy the indulgence and lose the guilt, but be prepared for a migraine.

Long Answer: Undoubtedly, there will be times—a celebratory meal out, a dinner with friends, a holiday meal with family—when you may dabble in forbidden foods. If this indulgence includes either wheat flour or a sugary treat, you will likely notice two things.

One, you will probably feel crummy (upset stomach, postmeal fatigue/sleepiness). No longer indulging in these items regularly, you will now fully appreciate the powerful impact they have on your physiology. And if you are one of the one in three (or more) who are gluten sensitive, you will feel downright *lousy*.

Two, there's a good chance you will end up with a migraine. So be prepared—make sure you've brought something along with you for migraine relief so you can catch it before it spirals out of control. Another option is to take a prophylactic dose of ibuprofen (400 to 600 mg) either immediately prior to or at the start of your "cheat meal." One of the upsides of eating this way is that you will find that abortive migraine medications work *much better* than they used to.

In all likelihood, provided these cheat meals are only an occasional indulgence, you'll be able to knock out the ensuing migraine readily. Just remember to be prepared so you can catch it early!

Will I lose weight eating like this?

Short Answer: Yes, most folks who stick to an ancestral diet will ultimately end up at their genetically-encoded ideal body fat composition.

Long Answer: The vast majority of folks who transition to this way of eating will lose weight. We humans accumulate excess body fat when we eat foods that are outside of our evolutionary experience. Just like it does with body temperature, mineral concentration, and fluid balance, our *hypothalamus* (which is what generates our feelings of hunger and satiety) is designed to maintain our body fat within a tight range for optimal function. And it's designed to do so *automatically*. Yet our hypothalamus is designed to maintain body-fat homeostasis with a particular set of foods—those that our species has adapted to during the past two million years. When we eat these evolutionarily appropriate foods, our body's natural mechanisms for body-fat regulation will maintain body fat within a very narrow range. This is true for every species in the animal kingdom (and is also why obesity is only a problem for animals we keep as pets or in zoos). It is only when we eat foods that are outside of our evolutionary experience that we subvert the hypothalamus's capacity to maintain an optimal percentage of body fat and begin to store unhealthy amounts of body fat.

So unless you are already at ideal body-fat composition, what will happen as you shed evolutionarily inappropriate foods is that your body will burn off excess body fat until you reach your optimal, genetically determined amount. To lose weight eating an ancestral diet all you must do is listen to your hypothalamus, which means eating when you're hungry and stopping when you're satisfied. There are no calories to be counted, no six-meals-a-day regimen to follow. When it comes to fat regulation, your hypothalamus is far smarter than you are.

My kids are very picky eaters. How can I get them eating like this?

Short Answer: Transition them slowly, and consult www.mymigraine miracle.com for kid-friendly recipes.

Long Answer: Without a doubt, it's far easier to maintain this way of eating if everyone else is eating this way, particularly if you're the one preparing the meals. You may also wish to transition your kids to a healthier way of eating. As a whole, kids today suffer from unprece-dented and catastrophic levels of obesity and diabetes, an epidemic that, not by coincidence, occurred in concert with an extraordinary rise in the consumption of sweetened beverages.

If you're fortunate enough to have kids who'll eat anything and simply have whatever you're having, then count your blessings, as your work is done. For the rest of you, transitioning your children to this way of eating may present a challenge. It is one worth taking on, for sure, as you'll be making a tremendous impact on their health that will be real-ized throughout the rest of their lives.

For kids, a stepwise approach affords the best chance of success. As a first step, eliminate sweetened beverages (sodas and any others with sugar in the list of ingredients) and processed foods. Then determine all the foods that they currently eat that meet the guidelines set out in chapter 5. If you can create a full menu using these items, then these can become the mainstays of their diet over time. If not, then you will need to introduce some new items into their diet. Fortunately, many others have been down this road, and lots of folks have created innova-tive ways to make an ancestral diet "kid-friendly." Personally, I have children ages five and eight, and my oldest is a very "selective" eater. Yet nowadays both my kids eat this way roughly 95 percent of the time and fully enjoy their meals. Visit www.mymigrainemiracle.com to find recipes for several of our favorite kid-friendly snacks and meals.

I've been following the guidelines diligently but am still getting the occasional migraine. What might be the problem?

Short Answer: Look for hidden ingredients that could be sabotaging your efforts; try a couple weeks of a very low-carbohydrate, ketogenic diet; consider taking a nutritional supplement; and make sure any mental health needs are being addressed.

Long Answer: If you've been diligently following all of the guidelines laid out in chapter 5 and are still experiencing the occasional headache (assuming these aren't occurring after a cheat meal), then do the following:

1. Scrutinize the foods you eat to make sure nothing nefarious has snuck into the food you're eating. Read all labels to look for unwanted ingredients—it's astonishing how many foods have either sugar or wheat flour added to them.

2. If you do not find any potential suspects after step one, then try reducing your daily carbohydrate consumption to between 20 to 50 grams per day for a period of at least two weeks. The goal here is to ramp up the production of *ketone bodies* in the brain. To be sure that you're producing significant amounts of ketone bodies, you can use ketostix (available online or at the drug store), which can detect the presence of ketones in the urine. If ketones are present in the urine, then you can be assured adequate amounts are reaching the brain as well and providing extra protection against migraines.

    If the two-week ketogenic diet works, then you can try slowly increasing your carbohydrate consumption at any point after the two-week period, if you desire. If migraines resurface, then return to the very low-carbohydrate, ketogenic approach.

3. If migraines still occur after two weeks in ketosis, then try adding in one of the nutritional supplements that have been shown to reduce migraine frequency. As discussed in chapter 2, this includes magnesium, vitamin B2 (riboflavin), and

butterbur. You can add in one at a time, or you can try them in combination. Migrelief, a combination supplement available over the counter (best found online), contains two of these (magnesium and vitamin B2) in one pill for convenience.

4. If you've been through all of these steps and are still experiencing headaches, make sure you're paying attention to mental health needs. While some folks experience anxiety and depression overtly, for others it may manifest largely as physical symptoms, including headaches. And if these issues aren't addressed directly, they can sabotage even your best efforts at controlling your migraines.

   Lastly, if you find your headaches resistant to multiple approaches, it is certainly worth discussing with your doctor. In very rare cases, treatment-resistant headaches can be a sign of pathology inside the skull.

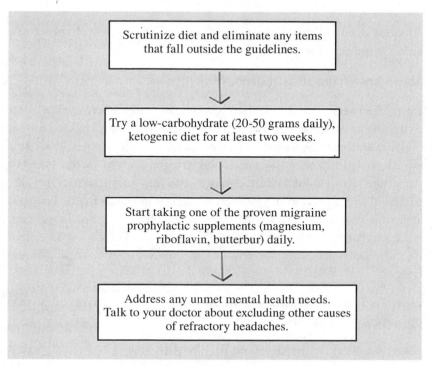

Table 1 - A stepwise approach for addressing persistent migraines.

My migraines have disappeared except during menstruation. What can I do about these?

Short Answer: Consider a very low-carbohydrate (20–50 g daily), ketogenic diet starting three to five days prior to until the end of menstruation for added migraine protection.

Long Answer: For women, if there's any time when the migraine beast may still rear its ugly head in spite of adherence to an ancestral diet, it is during menstruation. The occasional woman may find herself still experiencing headaches during this period of time. Fortunately, as discussed above, the headache should remain very sensitive to abortive medication. For those who wish to eliminate these altogether, first try supplementing with magnesium, riboflavin, or butterbur during menstruation. If migraines continue in spite of these measures, then reduce dietary carbohydrate to between 20 to 50 milligrams per day beginning three to five days before the anticipated start of menstruation, continuing until the completion of menses.

Alcohol used to be a big trigger for me. Is there any chance I can enjoy it again in moderation?

Short Answer: In all likelihood, yes.

Long Answer: One of the things you will likely experience after switching to an ancestral diet is that some of the foods that once were major migraine triggers for you have lost some of their potency, including alcohol. If alcohol has been a big trigger for you in the past but you'd like to still enjoy it in moderation, you may find yourself now able to slowly add it back in moderation with no untoward effects. Just wait at least a few weeks after your transition to try doing so. In general, wine and spirits are less problematic than beer, as the gluten contained in most beers (though the amount is small) presents an additional trigger.

How do I maintain this way of eating on long car trips? My only options are fast food!

Short Answer: Be prepared and pack healthy snacks before you leave.

Long Answer: Adhering to an ancestral diet while traveling, particularly for long distances in the car, presents another unique challenge. Gone are the quick gas station runs for crackers and soda, or a burger and fries at McDonald's, that are the mainstay of road-trip cuisine. Once again, to manage these excursions successfully, a bit of advance planning is in order. If you're traveling with a cooler, try packing some deli meats, cheese, and possibly some olives to make the Meat and Cheese Roll-Ups from chapter 6. Nuts with or without dried fruit also make a great snack for long car trips. Dried meats (i.e., jerky) are also another great option that don't require refrigeration. You can make these yourself or purchase from a natural-foods store (not the kind you can get at the gas station).

If you do find yourself with no other options but drive-through fast food, either find something on the menu that's largely diet-compliant (salad with chicken, for example) or that can be modified to be so (e.g., take the bun off the burger, etc.).

Won't eating like this raise my cholesterol?

Short Answer: Yes—the good kind. Those who switch from a typical Western diet to an ancestral one will experience a lowering of triglycerides; substantial elevation in HDL, or "good," cholesterol; modest elevation in LDL, or "bad," cholesterol (due to an increase in particle size, which is a good thing); and a resultant increase in the HDL:LDL ratio (a very good thing).

Long Answer: When it comes to the shortcomings of mainstream health authorities, the oversimplification and misinformation proffered on the subject of blood cholesterol and heart disease stands as one of the largest. Whenever I first broach the subject of cholesterol with my patients, I find that the vast majority of them are under the impression that 1) high blood cholesterol leads to heart disease, and 2) high blood cholesterol is caused by eating too much cholesterol. They are often shocked to find out that neither of these things is true. Women over the age of 55 are also often surprised to learn that, for them, lower blood cholesterol raises their risk of dying (Emond and Zareba 1997)!

The truth about cholesterol and its relationship to the hardening of the arteries (atherosclerosis) that leads to stroke and heart disease is actually far more nuanced and complex than what's typically presented.

Furthermore, our understanding of cholesterol and its relationship to atherosclerosis has changed markedly during the past couple of decades, and many of the details are still unknown.

First of all, cholesterol is necessary for life. It is not some nefarious substance floating around in your blood just to promote your early demise but rather an essential structural component of every cell in the body and a necessary ingredient in the synthesis of several hormones and vitamins. Second, it is not cholesterol itself that leads to atherosclerosis, but rather cholesterol-carrying *particles* known as *low-density lipoproteins* (LDL) that end up getting stuck inside the arterial walls, ultimately leading to the formation of the plaques whose rupture causes heart attack and stroke. Folks who have lots of very small, oxidized LDL particles and high levels of serum triglycerides are at the highest risk of forming these artery-clogging plaques (Cromwell et al. 2007; Meisinger 2005 et al.). What's the quickest way to generate lots of very small, oxidized LDL particles and high triglycerides in your bloodstream? Eat lots of sugar (Stanhope et al. 2011).

An ancestral diet, being low in sugar and high in good fats, leads to elevation in high-density lipoprotein- (HDL-) associated cholesterol (the "good" cholesterol, using the unfortunate lexicon of today), lowering of serum triglycerides, and the transformation of LDL particles from small, oxidized, artery-invading gremlins to large, buoyant, and non-atherogenic particles.

I'm a vegetarian. Is it possible to eat like this without eating meat?

Short Answer: Yes, perhaps with a few compromises.

Long Answer: If you don't presently eat meat, you may wonder if it's possible to maintain this restriction while still reaping the migraine protection afforded by an ancestral diet. I can relate to your position, as I was a vegetarian at one point in my life, largely out of concerns regarding the ethical treatment of livestock. The major challenge you will face in maintaining an evolutionarily appropriate vegetarian diet will be finding an adequate source of dietary protein. If you end up eating less protein than your body requires, your body will begin to break down its own lean tissue (muscle first) in order to meet that need—an unhealthy outcome.

If you are open to eating and can easily tolerate high-fat dairy (i.e., not lactose-intolerant or casein-allergic) and eggs, then these items can meet most of that need (whole milk, Greek yogurt, cheese, etc.). You'll just need to pay attention to make sure you're getting enough protein in your diet. In general, if you are sedentary (which hopefully you aren't), your protein intake in grams per day should be about 40 percent of your ideal body weight (56 g for a 140-pound person, for example). Moderately active individuals (exercising several times per week) should aim for around 60 percent of ideal body weight. Very active individuals (high-level athletes, those involved in strength training, etc.) should aim for around 80 percent of ideal body weight.

If dairy and eggs aren't a part of your diet, then the level of difficulty increases substantially. In general, most plants are low in protein, and the quantity of vegetable matter you'd need to consume to meet your protein needs would be impractical. A few vegetables, however, are reasonably protein dense. Soybeans are one, and are what many vegetarians and vegans use to meet their protein requirements. Yet soybeans were not a part of our preagricultural diet, and as such soy protein is recognized as a foreign substance by our immune system. Combine this with the fact that soy lectin disrupts the intestinal lining, and you have all the right conditions for diet-induced inflammatory and autoimmune disorders. Needless to say, meeting protein requirements with soy products is not an acceptable solution.

Legumes, a class of plant that includes beans and peas, are also comparatively high in protein, and so represent another potential vegetarian option to meet dietary protein needs. Like cereal grains, most legumes are toxic in their raw state and require processing before they can be eaten safely. As such, they were a negligible part of our preagricultural diet and may still exert deleterious effects on our health through their ability to disrupt the intestinal lining. I think they are fine in moderation, provided the other parts of your diet are in place, but I would be very reluctant to make them a dietary staple.

Nuts are another potential protein source, but once again the problem is one of quantity. Nuts are high in omega-6 fatty acids, which are pro-inflammatory. This poses little problem if you've removed other sources of excess omega-6 (vegetable and seed oils) unless you're eating a lot of them, which you would need to do if they were functioning as your primary protein source.

Quinoa has become the latest vegetarian protein source du jour. While not likely a meaningful part of our ancestors' diets, quinoa doesn't contain any potentially harmful components and it is nutritionally dense. One cup of it provides 8 grams of protein. As such, it represents perhaps the best source for vegetable protein, and conceivably could meet much of the protein needs for someone with a relatively low daily requirement.

As you can see, adhering to a vegetarian diet within the ancestral framework presents its challenges, particularly if dairy and eggs are not an option. Doing so will require some degree of compromise, but it is still an effort worth pursuing. Even if you are only able to remain mostly within the boundaries of an ancestral diet, you will still reap great health benefits, including enhanced protection against migraines.

Finally, if you're presently avoiding meat due to concerns about animal welfare, I'd urge you to at least consider the possibility of obtaining meat outside of the factory farming system. My decision to become a vegetarian was made largely over concerns about how factory-raised animals were treated. Nowadays, almost all of the meat I consume comes from animals raised humanely in their natural setting. I have visited the farms where my beef, chicken, and pork come from, and one of the farmers I buy from has become a good friend. I know firsthand that the animals there are well loved and cared for, and lead a peaceful and contented existence. I have no qualms eating animals raised in this manner and furthermore enjoy the opportunity to support the farmers who are making the effort to raise livestock sustainably and humanely. The more of us who support the farmers doing this important work, the better chance we have of creating a future where all animals are raised in a manner we can feel good about.

I only get a migraine every once in a while, but I get milder headaches quite frequently. Will this help for those?

Short Answer: Yes!

Long Answer: One of the most common misconceptions about migraines is that they always have to be severe, knock-down-drag-out episodes to qualify as a "real" migraine. This is not the case. A migraine headache with the full spectrum of associated features is just the most robust, extreme realization of the migraine process in the brain. This misconception about migraines has led to the corollary and no less widespread notion that migraines that are not severe must be something else entirely, in most cases labeled as "sinus" or "tension" headaches. Once again, this is not true. Almost every headache experienced by a migraineur, from the dull nagging aches to the debilitating head scorchers, is some variant of migraine. As such, you will find an ancestral diet to be an effective prophylactic against all variations of headache.

How long do I need to eat like this? If I go back to my old eating habits, will my migraines return?

Short Answer: The principles outlined in this book should guide your eating decisions for the rest of your life.

Long Answer: I consider the way of eating I've outlined here to be not only the best method for preventing migraines but also the best way to ensure optimum health and longevity. As such, I'd recommend you continue to eat this way for the rest of your life. And though the propensity to experience a migraine does decline with age to some extent, in all likelihood, if you revert back to your old eating habits, your health will decline, and your former pattern of migraines will return.

Recommended Reading and Additional Resources

Those of you who'd like to dig deeper into the world of ancestral health and nutrition, or those looking for additional resources to help you transition to this lifestyle, will be pleased to find a substantial and ever-expanding number of resources at your disposal. During the past decade, the ancestral health movement has grown at an incredible pace, fueled by countless success stories from those who have reclaimed their health, reversed chronic illnesses, and enjoyed newfound wellness and vitality. It is a movement that has grown in leaps and bounds in spite of sometimes vocal opposition by mainstream health figures, buttressed by its irrefutable results and solid scientific framework. The proof, as they say, is in the pudding.

Here is a small sampling of some of my favorite print and web resources on ancestral health:

ON THE WEB

The Migraine Miracle website. The companion website for this book, located at www.mymigrainemiracle.com, contains a host of additional resources for migraine sufferers, including a continually updated section of recipes.

Mark's Daily Apple. Created by *Primal Blueprint* author Mark Sisson and located at www.marksdailyapple.com, Mark's Daily Apple is a wonderful resource for those who've adopted this way of eating. In addition to providing practical, well-written daily blog posts on a wide range of topics, this site is also a terrific source for recipes that are well within the guidelines outlined in *The Migraine Miracle.*

Blog of Michael and Mary Dan Eades, M.D. Located at www .proteinpower.com, this is the blog of freethinking physicians who have been successfully treating patients with low-carbohydrate diets, ancestral-style diets, and challenging nutritional dogma for years. Lots of thoughtful analysis, commentary, and advice.

BOOKS

The Primal Blueprint by Mark Sisson (Primal Nutrition Inc., 2012). A popular, easily accessible book on the benefits of a "primal" diet and lifestyle—and a fun read. Mark's follow-up book, *The Primal Connection*, further explores how reconnecting with ancient ways of living in our increasingly fast-paced, distraction-laden world enhances our mental and spiritual health.

Good Calories, Bad Calories (Random House, 2008) by Gary Taubes. An exhaustive, meticulously-researched account of why so much of what we've been led to believe about nutrition is wrong, and how it all happened. As much a story about diet and health as it is the precarious nature of good science, it may one day be regarded as the spark that ignited a paradigm shift. It should be required reading for anyone in the field of health or science in general. Taubes's follow-up book, *Why We Get Fat*, is sometimes referred to as the lighter version of *Good Calories, Bad Calories*, and perhaps better suited for those less interested in scientific detail.

Food and Western Disease (Wiley-Blackwell 2010) by Staffan Lindeberg. Authored by professor Staffan Lindeberg, who has spent a good chunk of his professional career directly studying the health of several indigenous peoples, *Food and Western Disease* is an exhaustively researched, rigorous work that explores the health of hunter-gatherer societies and potential mechanisms by which modern diets cause the diseases of civilization.

ARTICLES

Blouet, C., G. J. Schwartz. 2010. "Hypothalamic Nutrient Sensing in the Control of Energy Homeostasis." *Behavioural Brain Research* 209(1): 1–12.

Cassidy, C. M. 1980. "Nutrition and Health in Agriculturalists and Hunter-Gatherers: A Case Study of Two Prehistoric Populations." In *Nutritional Anthropology,* edited by N. W. Jerome et al. Pleasantville, NY: Redgrave Publishing Company.

Cordain, L., J. B. Miller, S. B. Eaton et al. 2000. "Plant-Animal Subsistence Ratios and Macronutrient Energy Estimations in Worldwide Hunter-Gatherer Diets." *The American Journal of Clinical Nutrition* 71(3): 682–92.

Cordain, L., S. B. Eaton, J. B. Miller et al. 2002. "The Paradoxical Nature of Hunter-Gatherer Diets: Meat-Based, Yet Non-Atherogenic." *The European Journal of Clinical Nutrition* 56 Suppl 1: S42–52.

Fasano, A. "Systemic Autoimmune Disorders in Celiac Disease." 2006. *Current Opinions in Gastroenterology* 22(6): 674–9.

Fouché, F. P. 1923. "Freedom of Negro Races from Cancer." *British Medical Journal* 3261: 1116.

Howard, B. V., L. Van Horn, J. Hsia et al. 2006. "Low-Fat Dietary Pattern and Risk of Cardiovascular Disease: The Women's Health Initiative Randomized Controlled Dietary Modification Trial." *Journal of the American Medical Association* 295(6): 655–66.

Ishkanian, G., H. Blumenthal, C. J. Webster et al. 2007. "Efficacy of Sumatriptan Tablets in Migraineurs Self-Described or Physician-Diagnosed as Having Sinus Headache: A Randomized, Double-Blind, Placebo-Controlled Study." *Clinical Therapeutics* 29(1): 99–109.

Jenkinson, A., M. F. Franklin, K. Wahle, et al. 1999. "Dietary Intakes of Polyunsaturated Fatty Acids and Indices of Oxidative Stress in Human Volunteers." *European Journal of Clinical Nutrition* 53(7): 523–8.

Kari, E., and J. M. DelGaudio. 2008. "Treatment of Sinus Headache as Migraine: The Diagnostic Utility of Triptans." *Laryngoscope* 118(12): 2235–9.

Kobak, K. A., D. J. Katzelnick, G. Sands et al. 2005. "Prevalence and Burden of Illness of Migraine in Managed Care Patients." *Journal of Managed Care Pharmacy* 11(2): 124–36.

Kowalski, L. M., and J. Bujko. 2012. "Evaluation of Biological and Clinical Potential of Paleolithic Diet." *Roczniki Państwowego Zakładu Higieny* 63(1): 9–15. Original article in Polish.

Kratz, M., T. Baars, and S. Guyenet. 2013. "The Relationship Between High-Fat Dairy Consumption and Obesity, Cardiovascular, and Metabolic Disease." *European Journal of Nutrition* 52(1): 1–24.

Lammert, F., and D. Q. Wang. 2005. "New Insights into the Genetic Regulation of Intestinal Cholesterol Absorption." *Gastroenterology* 129(2): 718–34.

Leone, M., A. Franzini, A. P. Cecchini et al. 2010. "Hypothalamic Deep Brain Stimulation in the Treatment of Chronic Cluster Headache." *Therapeutic Advances in Neurological Disorders* 3(3): 187–95.

MacGregor, E. A., J. Brandes, A. Eikermann et al. 2004. "Impact of Migraine on Patients and Their Families: The Migraine and Zolmitriptan Evaluation (MAZE) Survey—Phase III." *Current Medical Research and Opinion* 20(7): 1143–50. Erratum in: *Current Medical Research and Opinion.* 20(10): 1689.

Maggioni, F., M. Margoni, and G. Zanchin. 2011. "Ketogenic Diet in Migraine Treatment: A Brief but Ancient History." *Cephalalgia* 31(10): 1150–1.

Moncrieff, J., S. Wessely, and R. Hardy. 2004. "Active Placebos Versus Antidepressants for Depression." *Cochrane Database of Systematic Reviews* (1):CD003012.

Richards, M. P. 2002. "A Brief Review of the Archaeological Evidence for Palaeolithic and Neolithic Subsistence." *European Journal of Clinical Nutrition* 56(12): 16 p following 1262.

Rose, G. A., W. B. Thomson, and R. T. Williams. 1965. "Corn Oil in Treatment of Ischaemic Heart Disease." *British Medical Journal.* 1(5449): 1531–3.

Sadur, C. N., and R. H. Eckel. 1982. "Insulin Stimulation of Adipose Tissue Lipoprotein Lipase: Use of the Euglycemic Clamp Technique." *Journal of Clinical Investigation* 69(5): 1119–25.

Santos, F. L., S. S. Esteves, A. da Costa Pereira et al. 2012. "Systematic Review and Meta-Analysis of Clinical Trials of the Effects of Low-Carbohydrate Diets on Cardiovascular Risk Factors." *Obesity Review* 13(11): 1048–66.

Schweitzer, A. Trans. A. B. Lemke. 1998. *Out of Life and Thought: An Autobiography.* Baltimore: Johns Hopkins University Press. (Originally published 1933).

Shai, I., D. Schwarzfuchs, Y. Henkin et al. 2008. "Weight Loss with a Low-Carbohydrate, Mediterranean, or Low-Fat Diet." *New England Journal of Medicine* 359(3): 229–41.

Storrs, C. 2011. "Will a Gluten-Free Diet Improve Your Health?" *CNN Health.* www.cnn.com/2011/HEALTH/04/12/gluten.free. diet.improve/index.html, accessed January 7, 2013.

Tfelt-Hansen, P., P. De Vries, and P. R. Saxena. 2000. "Triptans in Migraine: A Comparative Review of Pharmacology, Pharmacokinetics and Efficacy." *Drugs* 60(6): 1259–87.

Tseng, M., R. A. Breslow, B. I. Graubard et al. 2005. "Dairy, Calcium, and Vitamin D Intakes and Prostate Cancer Risk in the National Health and Nutrition Examination Epidemiologic Follow-Up Study Cohort." *The American Journal of Clinical Nutrition* 81(5): 1147–54.

References

Abdelmalek, M. F., A. Suzuki, C. Guy et al. 2010. "Increased Fructose Consumption Is Associated with Fibrosis Severity in Patients with Nonalcoholic Fatty Liver Disease." *Hepatology* 51(6): 1961–71.

Anderson, J. 2012. "How Many People Have Gluten Sensitivity?" *Celiac Disease and Gluten Sensitivity*. http://celiacdisease.about.com/od/gluten intolerance/a/How-Many-People-Have-Gluten-Sensitivity.htm, accessed January 10, 2013.

Angel, J. L. 1984. "Health as a Crucial Factor in the Changes from Hunting to Developed Farming in the Eastern Mediterranean." In *Paleopathology at the Origins of Agriculture*, edited by M. N. Cohen and G. J. Armelagos. London: Academic Press.

Barber, S. C. and P. J. Shaw. 2010. "Oxidative Stress in ALS: Key Role in Motor Neuron Injury and Therapeutic Target." *Free Radical Biology and Medicine* 48(5): 629–41.

Boyd, D. B. 2003. "Insulin and Cancer." *Integrative Cancer Therapies* 2(4): 315–29.

Brehm, B. J., R. J. Seeley, S. R. Daniels et al. 2003. "A Randomized Trial Comparing a Very Low Carbohydrate Diet and a Calorie-Restricted Low Fat Diet on Body Weight and Cardiovascular Risk Factors in Healthy Women." *The Journal of Clinical Endocrinology and Metabolism* 88(4): 1617–23.

Cai, D. and T. Liu. 2011. "Hypothalamic Inflammation: A Double-Edged Sword to Nutritional Diseases." *Annals of the New York Academy of Sciences* 1243:(1) E1–39.

Cai, D. and T. Liu. 2012. "Inflammatory Cause of Metabolic Syndrome via Brain Stress and NF-kB." *Aging* (Albany, N.Y.) 4(2): 98–115.

Carpay, J., J. Schoenen, F. Ahmad et al. 2004. "Efficacy and Tolerability of Sumatriptan Tablets in a Fast-Disintegrating, Rapid-Release Formulation for the Acute Treatment of Migraine: Results of a Multicenter,

Randomized, Placebo-Controlled Study." *Clinical Therapeutics* 26(2): 214–23.

Chajès, V., A. C. Thiébaut, M. Rotival et al. 2008. "Association Between Serum Trans-Monounsaturated Fatty Acids and Breast Cancer Risk in the E3N-EPIC Study." *American Journal of Epidemiology* 167(11): 1312–20.

Cho, E., S. A. Smith-Warner, D. Spiegelman et al. 2004. "Dairy Foods, Calcium, and Colorectal Cancer: A Pooled Analysis of 10 Cohort Studies." *Journal of the National Cancer Institute* 96(13): 1015–22. Erratum in: *Journal of the National Cancer Institute.* 2004 96(22): 1724.

Cohen, M. N. and G. J. Armelagos. 1984. *Paleopathology at the Origins of Agriculture.* London: Academic Press.

Cordain, L. 1999. "Cereal Grains: Humanity's Double-Edged Sword." *World Review of Nutrition and Dietetics.* 84: 19–73.

Cordain, L., S. B. Eaton, A. Sebastian et al. 2005. "Origins and Evolution of the Western Diet: Health Implications for the 21st Century." *The American Journal of Clinical Nutrition* 81(2): 341–54.

Cosnes, J., C. Cellier, S. Viola et al. (Groupe D'Etude et de Recherche Sur la Maladie Coeliaque). 2008. "Incidence of Autoimmune Diseases in Celiac Disease: Protective Effect of the Gluten-Free Diet." *Clinical Gastroenterology and Hepatology* 6(7): 753–8.

Cromwell, W. C., J. D. Otvos, M. J. Keyes et al. 2007. "LDL Particle Number and Risk of Future Cardiovascular Disease in the Framingham Offspring Study—Implications for LDL Management." *Journal of Clinical Lipidology* 1(6): 583–92.

Dayton, S. and M. L. Pearce. 1969. "Diet High in Unsaturated Fat: A Controlled Clinical Trial." *Minnesota Medicine* 52(8): 1237–42.

Denuelle, M., N. Fabre, P. Payoux et al. 2007. "Hypothalamic Activation in Spontaneous Migraine Attacks." *Headache* 47(10): 1418–26.

Diez-Gonzalez, F., T. R. Callaway, M. G. Kizoulis et al. 1998. "Grain Feeding and the Dissemination of Acid-Resistant *Escherichia Coli* from Cattle." *Science* 281(5383): 1666–8.

Emond, M. J. and W. Zareba. 1997. "Prognostic Value of Cholesterol in Women of Different Ages." *Journal of Women's Health* 6(3): 295–307.

Fairfield, K. M., D. J. Hunter, G. A. Colditz et al. 2004. "A Prospective Study of Dietary Lactose and Ovarian Cancer." *International Journal of Cancer* 110(2): 271–7.

Frantz Jr., I. D., E. A. Dawson, P. L. Ashman et al. 1989. "Test of Effect of Lipid Lowering by Diet on Cardiovascular Risk: The Minnesota Coronary Survey." *Arteriosclerosis, Thrombosis, and Vascular Biology* 9(1): 129–35.

Gallai, V., P. Sarchielli, G. Coata et al. 1992. "Serum and Salivary Magnesium Levels in Migraine: Results in a Group of Juvenile Patients." *Headache* 32(3): 132–5.

Gardner, C. D., A. Kiazand, S. Alhassan et al. 2007. "Comparison of the Atkins, Zone, Ornish, and LEARN Diets for Change in Weight and Related Risk Factors Among Overweight Premenopausal Women: The A to Z Weight Loss Study: A Randomized Trial." *Journal of the American Medical Association* 297(9): 969–77. Erratum in: *Journal of the American Medical Association.* 2007. 298(2): 178.

Gasior, M., M. A. Rogawski, and A. L. Hartman. 2006. "Neuroprotective and Disease-Modifying Effects of the Ketogenic Diet." *Behavioural Pharmacology* 17(5-6): 431–9.

Hermanussen, M., and F. Poustka. 2003. "Stature of Early Europeans." *Hormones* 2(3): 175–8.

Holland, S., S. D. Silberstein, F. Freitag et al. 2012. "Evidence-Based Guideline Update—NSAIDs and Other Complementary Treatments for Episodic Migraine Prevention in Adults: Report of the Quality Standards Subcommittee of the American Academy of Neurology and the American Headache Society." *Neurology* 78(17): 1346–53.

Holvoet, P. 2004. "Oxidized LDL and Coronary Heart Disease." *Acta Cardiologica* 59(5): 479–84.

Holvoet, P., A. Mertens, P. Verhamme et al. 2001. "Circulating Oxidized LDL Is a Useful Marker for Identifying Patients with Coronary Artery Disease." *Arteriosclerosis, Thrombosis, and Vascular Biology* 21(5): 844–8.

Hrdlicka, A. 1908. *Physiological and Medical Observations Among the Indians of Southwestern United States and Northern Mexico.* Washington D.C.: U.S. Government Printing Office.

Hutton, S. K. 1925. *Health Conditions and Disease Incidence Among the Eskimos of Labrador.* London: Wessex Press.

Jackson, J. R., W. W. Eaton, N. G. Cascella et al. 2012. "Neurologic and Psychiatric Manifestations of Celiac Disease and Gluten Sensitivity." *The Psychiatric Quarterly* 83(1): 91–102.

Kneepkens, C. M. and B. M. von Blomberg. 2012. "Clinical Practice: Coeliac Disease." *European Journal of Pediatrics* 171(7): 1011–21.

Larsson, S. C., L. Bergkvist, and A. Wolk. 2004. "Milk and Lactose Intakes and Ovarian Cancer Risk in the Swedish Mammography Cohort." *The American Journal of Clinical Nutrition* 80(5): 1353–7.

Larsson, S. C., L. Bergkvist, and A. Wolk. 2005. "High-Fat Dairy Food and Conjugated Linoleic Acid Intakes in Relation to Colorectal Cancer Incidence in the Swedish Mammography Cohort." *The American Journal of Clinical Nutrition* 82(4): 894–900.

Levin, I. 1910. "Cancer Among the North American Indians and Its Bearing upon the Ethonological Distribution of Disease." *Zeitschrift fur Krebsforschung* 9(3): 422–35.

Lim, J. S., M. Mietus-Snyder, A. Valente et al. 2010. "The Role of Fructose in the Pathogenesis of NAFLD and the Metabolic Syndrome." *Nature Reviews: Gastroenterology and Hepatology* 7(5): 251–64.

Lindeberg, Staffan. 2010. *Food and Western Disease.* West Sussex, UK: Wiley-Blackwell.

Lipton, R. B., M. E. Bigal, M. Diamond et al. (AMPP Advisory Group) 2007. "Migraine Prevalence, Disease Burden, and the Need for Preventive Therapy." *Neurology* 68(5):343–9.

Lipton, R. B., H. Göbel, K. M. Einhäupl et al. 2004. "Petasites Hybridus Root (Butterbur) Is an Effective Preventive Treatment for Migraine." *Neurology* 63(12): 2240–4.

Liu, H. and A. P. Heaney. 2011. "Refined Fructose and Cancer." *Expert Opinion on Therapeutic Targets* 15(9): 1049–59.

Maalouf, M., J. M. Rho, and M. P. Mattson. 2009. "The Neuroprotective Properties of Calorie Restriction, the Ketogenic Diet, and Ketone Bodies." *Brain Research Reviews* 59(2): 293–315.

Maillard-Lefebvre, H., E. Boulanger, M. Daroux et al. 2009. "Soluble Receptor for Advanced Glycation End Products: A New Biomarker in Diagnosis and Prognosis of Chronic Inflammatory Diseases." *Rheumatology* 48(10): 1190–6.

May, A., M. Leone, H. Boecke, et al. 2006. "Hypothalamic Deep Brain Stimulation in Positron Emission Tomography." *Journal of Neuroscience* 26(13): 3589–93.

Meisinger, C., J. Baumert, N. Khuseyinova et al. 2005. "Plasma Oxidized Low-Density Lipoprotein a Strong Predictor for Acute Coronary Heart Disease Events in Apparently Healthy, Middle-Aged Men from the General Population." *Circulation* 112(5): 651–7.

Miller, A., C. Stanton, J. Murphy et al. 2003. "Conjugated Linoleic Acid (CLA)-Enriched Milk Fat Inhibits Growth and Modulates CLA-Responsive Biomarkers in MCF-7 and SW480 Human Cancer Cell Lines." *The British Journal of Nutrition* 90(5): 877–85.

Molleson, T. 1994. "The Eloquent Bones of Abu Hureyra." *Scientific American* 271(2): 70–5.

Moorman, P. G. and P. D. Terry. 2004. "Consumption of Dairy Products and the Risk of Breast Cancer: A Review of the Literature." *The American Journal of Clinical Nutrition* 80(1): 5–14.

Mozaffarian, D., M. B. Katan, A. Ascherio et al. 2006. "Trans-Fatty Acids and Cardiovascular Disease." *New England Journal of Medicine* 354(15): 1601–13.

Münch, G., M. Gerlach, J. Sian et al. 1998. "Advanced Glycation End Products in Neurodegeneration: More Than Early Markers of Oxidative Stress?" *Annals of Neurology* 44(3 Suppl 1): S85–8.

Nelson, G. J., P. C. Schmidt, and D. S. Kelley. 1995. "Low-Fat Diets Do Not Lower Plasma Cholesterol Levels in Healthy Men Compared to High-Fat Diets with Similar Fatty Acid Composition at Constant Caloric Intake." *Lipids* 30(11): 969–76.

Olesen, J., and R. B. Lipton. 1994. "Migraine Classification and Diagnosis: International Headache Society Criteria." *Neurology* 44(6 Suppl 4): S6–10.

O'Shea, M., R. Devery, F. Lawless et al. 2000. "Milk Fat Conjugated Linoleic Acid (CLA) Inhibits Growth of Human Mammary MCF-7 Cancer Cells." *Anticancer Research* 20(5B): 3591–601.

Patel, A., P. L. Pyzik, Z. Turner, et al. 2010. "Long-Term Outcomes of Children Treated with the Ketogenic Diet in the Past." *Epilepsia* 51(7): 1277–82.

Ramsden, C. E., D. Zamora, B. Leelarthaepin et al. 2013. "Use of Dietary Linoleic Acid for Secondary Prevention of Coronary Heart Disease and Death: Evaluation of Recovered Data from the Sydney Diet Heart Study and Updated Meta-Analysis." *British Medical Journal* 346:e8707.

Rodrigo, L., C. Hernández-Lahoz, D. Fuentes et al. 2011. "Prevalence of Celiac Disease in Multiple Sclerosis." *BMC Neurology* 11(1): 31.

Rousset, H. 2004. "A Great Imitator for the Allergologist: Intolerance to Gluten." *European Annals of Allergy and Clinical Immunology* 36(3): 96–100.

Rubio-Tapia, A. and J. A. Murray. 2010. "Celiac Disease." *Current Opinions in Gastroenterology* 26(2): 116–22.

Samaha, F. F., N. Iqbal, P. Seshadri et al. 2003. "A Low-Carbohydrate as Compared with a Low-Fat Diet in Severe Obesity." *New England Journal of Medicine* 348(21): 2074–81.

Samaie, A., N. Asghari, R. Ghorbani et al. 2012. "Blood Magnesium Levels in Migraineurs Within and Between the Headache Attacks: A Case Control Study." *The Pan African Medical Journal* 11(1): 46.

Sándor, P. S. and J. Afra. 2005. "Nonpharmacologic Treatment of Migraine." *Current Pain and Headache Reports* 9(3): 202–5.

Schnabel, T. G. 1928. "An Experience with a Ketogenic Dietary in Migraine." *Annals of Internal Medicine* 2(4): 341–7.

Schoenen, J., J. Jacquy, and M. Lenaerts. 1998. "Effectiveness of High-Dose Riboflavin in Migraine Prophylaxis: A Randomized Controlled Trial." *Neurology* 50(2): 466–70.

Schreiber, C. P., S. Hutchinson, C. J. Webster et al. 2004. "Prevalence of Migraine in Patients with a History of Self-Reported or

217

Physician-Diagnosed 'Sinus' Headache." *Archives of Internal Medicine* 164(16): 1769–72.

Sheftell, F. D., C. G. Dahlöf, J. L. Brandes et al. 2005. "Two Replicate Randomized, Double-Blind, Placebo-Controlled Trials of the Time to Onset of Pain Relief in the Acute Treatment of Migraine with a Fast-Disintegrating/Rapid-Release Formulation of Sumatriptan Tablets." *Clinical Therapeutics* 27(4): 407–17.

Silberstein, S., R. Lipton, D. Dodick et al. 2009 "Topiramate Treatment of Chronic Migraine: A Randomized, Placebo-Controlled Trial of Quality of Life and Other Efficacy Measures." *Headache* 49(8): 1153–62.

Simopoulos, A. P. 2002. "The Importance of the Ratio of Omega-6/Omega-3 Essential Fatty Acids." *Biomedicine and Pharmacotherapy* 56(8): 365–79.

Siri-Tarino, P. W., Q. Sun, F. B. Hu et al. 2010. "Meta-Analysis of Prospective Cohort Studies Evaluating the Association of Saturated Fat with Cardiovascular Disease." *The American Journal of Clinical Nutrition* 91(3):535-46.

Siri-Tarino, P. W., Q. Sun, F. B. Hu et al. 2010. "Saturated Fat, Carbohydrate, and Cardiovascular Disease." *The American Journal of Clinical Nutrition* 91(3): 502–9.

Smith, B. W. and L. A. Adams. 2011. "Non-Alcoholic Fatty Liver Disease." *Critical Reviews in Clinical Laboratory Sciences* 48(3): 97–113.

Snowder, G. D., L. D. Van Vleck, L. V. Cundiff et al. 2006. "Bovine Respiratory Disease in Feedlot Cattle: Environmental, Genetic, and Economic Factors." *Journal of Animal Science* 84(8): 1999–2008.

Song, K. S. and J. R. Choi. 2004. "Tissue Transglutaminase Autoantibodies in Patients with IgM Rheumatoid Factors." *Yonsei Medical Journal* 45(5): 960–2.

Srikanth, V., A. Maczurek, T. Phan et al. 2011. "Advanced Glycation Endproducts and Their Receptor RAGE in Alzheimer's Disease." *Neurobiology of Aging* 32(5): 763–77.

Stafstrom, C. E. and J. M. Rho. 2012. "The Ketogenic Diet as a Treatment Paradigm for Diverse Neurological Disorders." *Frontiers in Pharmacology* 3: 59.

Stanhope, K. L., A. A. Bremer, V. Medici et al. 2011. "Consumption of Fructose and High Fructose Corn Syrup Increase Postprandial Triglycerides, LDL-Cholesterol, and Apolipoprotein-B in Young Men and Women." *Journal of Clinical Endocrinology and Metabolism* 96(10): E1596–605.

Stanhope, K. L. and P. J. Havel. 2008. "Fructose Consumption: Potential Mechanisms for Its Effects to Increase Visceral Adiposity and Induce Dyslipidemia and Insulin Resistance." *Current Opinion in Lipidology* 19(1): 16–24.

Stender, S. and J. Dyerberg. 2004. "Influence of Trans-fatty Acids on Health." *Annals of Nutrition and Metabolism* 48(2): 61–6.

Strahlman, R. S. 2006. "Can Ketosis Help Migraine Sufferers? A Case Report." *Headache* 46(1): 182.

Tappy, L. 2012. "Q&A: 'Toxic' Effects of Sugar: Should We Be Afraid of Fructose?" *BMC Biology* 10(1): 42.

Taubes, G. 2008. *Good Calories, Bad Calories.* New York: Random House.

Taubes, G. 2011. "Is Sugar Toxic?" *New York Times Magazine.*

Tepper, S. J. 2004. "New Thoughts on Sinus Headache." *Allergy and Asthma Proceedings* 25(2): 95–6.

Tepper, S. J., C. G. Dahlöf, A. Dowson et al. 2004. "Prevalence and Diagnosis of Migraine in Patients Consulting Their Physician with a Complaint of Headache: Data from the Landmark Study." *Headache* 44(9): 856–64.

Trowell, H. C. and D. P. Burkitt, eds. 1981. *Western Diseases: Their Emergence and Prevention.* London: Edward Arnold.

Urbizu, A., E. Cuenca-León, M. Raspall-Chaure et al. 2010. "Paroxysmal Exercise-Induced Dyskinesia, Writer's Cramp, Migraine with Aura and Absence Epilepsy in Twin Brothers with a Novel SLC2A1 Missense Mutation." *Journal of the Neurological Sciences* 15;295(1-2): 110–3.

USDA Office of Communications. 2003. *Agriculture Fact Book.* Washington D.C.: U.S. Government Printing Office.

Varkey, E., A. Cider, J. Carlsson et al. 2011. "Exercise as Migraine Prophylaxis: A Randomized Study Using Relaxation and Topiramate as Controls." *Cephalalgia* 31(14): 1428–38.

Volek, J., M. Sharman, A. Gómez et al. 2004. "Comparison of Energy-Restricted Very Low-Carbohydrate and Low-Fat Diets on Weight Loss and Body Composition in Overweight Men and Women." *Nutrition and Metabolism* 1(1): 13.

Westman, E. C., W. S. Yancy Jr., J. C. Mavropoulos et al. 2008. "The Effect of a Low-Carbohydrate, Ketogenic Diet Versus a Low-Glycemic Index Diet on Glycemic Control in Type 2 Diabetes Mellitus." *Nutrition and Metabolism* 5: 36.

Yaffe, K., K. Lindquist, A. V. Schwartz et al. 2011. "Advanced Glycation End Product Level, Diabetes, and Accelerated Cognitive Aging." *Neurology* 77(14): 1351–6.

Yancy Jr., W. S., M. K. Olsen, J. R. Guyton et al. 2004. "A Low-Carbohydrate, Ketogenic Diet Versus a Low-Fat Diet to Treat Obesity and Hyperlipidemia: A Randomized, Controlled Trial." *Annals of Internal Medicine* 140(10): 769–77.

Josh Turknett, MD, is a 2001 graduate of the Emory School of Medicine, a board-certified neurologist, and a clinical researcher in the areas of migraine, stroke, Alzheimer's disease, and Parkinson's disease. Turknett maintains a busy neurology practice in Atlanta, GA, and has been recognized twice by www.vitals.com as one of America's most compassionate doctors. He lives in the metro Atlanta area with his wife Jenny, their two children, and an ever-expanding collection of banjos.

Jenny Turknett has a background in baking, catering, and event planning. She currently works as a freelance food writer and restaurant critic for the *Atlanta Journal-Constitution*. She lives in the greater Atlanta, GA, area with her husband Josh, their two children, and an ever-expanding collection of kitchen gadgets.

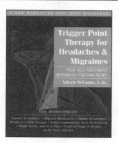
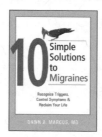
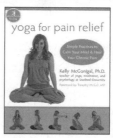
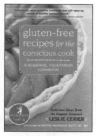
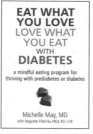
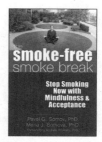